Green Smoothi

The Detox And Cleansing System to Lower Cholesterol and Glucose Levels, keeps You feeling Fuller For Longer, and Regulate Your Body's Cleansing Processes

Linda Pierce

Table of Contents

GREEN SMOOTHIES BIBLE I

INTRODUCTION 12

CHAPTER 1 15

WHAT ARE GREEN SMOOTHIES? 15

WHAT ARE GREEN SMOOTHIES 16

DAILY LIFE IMPROVEMENTS CAUSED BY GREEN SMOOTHIES AS BREAKFAST 16

Increases Your Daily Fruit & Vegetable Intake 17

Promotes weight reduction Naturally 17

Improves Hydration 18

Improves Digestion 18

Rejuvenates the body 19

Protects Against Free Radical Damage 19

Reliefs Symptoms of Depression 20

Better, & Clearer Skin 20

CHAPTER 2 22

GREEN SMOOTHIE HEALTH ADVANTAGES 22

Below are a Few of the Very Best Health Advantages of Green Smoothies:
.... 22

CHAPTER 3 32

GREEN SMOOTHIES 32

GREEN SMOOTHIES 33

Chlorophyll Rich 33

Helps to improve mental clarity and focus 33

Assists with digestion and overall metabolic function 34

Increases consumption of fruits & vegetables 34

Improves mood and helps fight depression 35

Promotes natural weight loss 35

Clearer skin 36

Hydration 36

Is Your Green Smoothie Vibrant? 37

Add more greens 37

Use low glycemic fruit 39

Make use of supplements! But make certain they're clean 40

Switch it up frequently and mindfully 42

CHAPTER 4 45

Immune Boosting Smoothies for Breakfast 45

Squeeze in a few lemons 45

Spa Smoothie 46

Pack in those greens 47

Acai Green 48

Coconut Turmeric Cream 49

CHAPTER 5 52

History of The Green Smoothie 52

Tips to make Green Smoothies 57

A view on avocados and fat content 59

Suggested Superfoods 61

Blueberries 62

Blue-green algae 62

Brazil nuts 62

Cacao 63

Coconut 63

Guava 63

Maca 63

Mesquite Powder 64

Pomegranate 65

Raspberries 65

Spirulina 65

Wheatgrass 65

Should You Buy or Make Your Milk? 66

How to make your milk 67

CHAPTER 6 69

SET OF FAT-BURNING FOODS AND USING SMOOTHIES FOR WEIGHT LOSS 69

    Apples 69

    Beets 70

    Broccoli 70

    Blackberries 70

    Cabbage 71

    Cantaloupe 71

    Carrots 71

    Celery 71

    Cherries 72

    Chives 72

    Cranberries 72

    Cucumbers 72

    Dandelion greens 73

    Goji berries 73

    Grape fruit 73

    Green beans 73

    Honeydew melon 74

    Juniper berries 74

    Kale 74

    Lettuce 74

    Lemons 75

    Limes 75

    Mango 75

    Nectarine 75

    Oatmeal 75

    Orange 76

    Papaya 76

    Peaches 76

    Pears 76

    Pineapple 76

    Pumpkin seeds 77

Raspberries 77

Spinach 77

Strawberries 77

Tomato 78

Watermelon 78

OTHER FRUITS AND VEGETABLES AND THEIR VITAMINS AND MINERALS 78

OTHER GREEN SMOOTHIE GREENS 81

Collard greens 81

Mustard greens 81

Rocket or arugula lettuce 81

Romaine lettuce 82

Swiss chard leaves 82

Turnip greens 82

Watercress 82

CHAPTER 7 84

CHOOSING YOUR GREENS 84

STORAGE AND USE FOR SMOOTHIES 84

OTHER ESSENTIALS 85

DRYING YOUR GREENS 86

STORING YOUR GREENS...86

STEMS..87

WHY GREEN FOODS?..87

Protein...88

Chlorophyll and blood-building properties.............................89

Calcium..89

Unequaled nutritional profile 90

Fiber 91

WAY TO SAVE MONEY ON GREEN SMOOTHIE 93

Figure out how to Garden 94

Choose Large Freezer 94

Harvest Edible Weeds...95

Buy in Bulk..96

Shop at Health Food Stores 96

Freeze fruit 96

Freeze Fresh Greens 97

Buy Frozen Spinach 97

Support Local Growers 97

Be familiar with small markets locally 97

CHAPTER 8 ....**99**

GREENGROCERY.. 99

Traditional Greens/Lettuces 99

Tops of root vegetables 100

Sea Vegetables... 101

Weeds 101

Sprouts 101

Herbs 102

FRUITS FOR GREEN SMOOTHIES 102

CHAPTER 9 ....**107**

GREEN SMOOTHIES RECIPES... 107

Cashew Blast.. 107

Yogurt with Cinnamon 107

Peanuts with Mint and Honey 108

Kiwi Guava Burst... 108

Spinach Surprise.. 109

Lychee with Eggs and Honey.. 110

Almond and Banana 110

Lettuce with Yogurt and Orange.................................... 111

Pear and Banana Blast.. 111

Banana Berry Smoothie 112

Strawberry with Lemonade.. 113

The Glowing Smoothie 113

Fight to become Well Smoothie 114

Powder of Green Smoothie 115

Renewal Smoothie 116

Greeny Green- Beginner's Luck 117

Cilantro with Mango Detox 118

Banana-Choc-Chai Smoothie 118

Banana Raspberry Yum 119

Berrylicious 120

Pineapple Broccoli Sensation..121

Pineapple Dilly Dally 121

Herbal Ginger Beet 122

Saladicious...123

Salad Sunset 125

Blue Bat 125

Blueberry Pineapple Smoothie 126

Berry Packed Smoothie 127

Just what A Lovely Pear..127

Tangy Tex Mex 128

Dance towards the Beet..129

Mango Spice...129

Choc-Mango Spice..130

Blue Eyes Smoothie 131

Vanilla Pudding Smoothie 132

Carob Vanilla Spice Pudding Smoothie.....................................133

Mint Vanilla Pudding Smoothie 134

Kiwi Vanilla Smoothie...135

Gleaming Green Spinach and Lettuce Smoothie 136

Vigour Booster Spinach and Collard Greens..............................138

Minty Papaya Green Smoothie 139

Green Piña Colada Smoothie...140

Kiwi Green Smoothie 142

Minty Green Smoothie 143

Avocado Lime Smoothie 144

Tropical Kale Green Smoothie 146

Almond Swirl 147

Aztec Chili Cacao 149

Berries 'n' Cream 150

Celery Green Smoothie...150

Collard Green smoothie..150

Mango Green Smoothie 151

Spicy Delicious Green Smoothie 151

All-Purpose Green Smoothie 152

Green tea extract Smoothie 152

Lemon Cucumber Green Smoothie 152

Cashew Green Smoothie 153

Orange Green Smoothie 153

Fruit and Green Smoothie 154

Ginger Green Smoothie.. 154

Melon Green Shake 155

Almond Coconut Yogurt Green Smoothie 155

Refreshing Green Smoothie 156

Banana Swiss Chard Smoothie with Lime 157

Spinach and Flaxseed Protein Smoothie 157

Mint Chocolate Smoothie with Spinach 158

Strawberry Banana Protein Smoothie with Spinach 159

Apple Cinnamon Smoothie with Romaine Lettuce 159

Green Peanut Butter and Banana Smoothie 160

Protein Pear and Kale Smoothie 160

Mint and Pear Smoothie with Ginger 161

Green Grape and Pumpkin Smoothie 162

Fruity Green Smoothie 162

Mean Greeny Juice 163

Veggie Smoothie 163

Grass of Apple 164

Grass of Wheat 165

Grass of Orange 165

Wintergreen smoothie 165

Spring with Green Smoothie 166

Summer with Green Smoothie 167

Fall in love Smoothie 167

Carrot with Spinach 168

Spinach with Tomato..169

Spinach with Beet Carrot..169

Cucumber and Spinach mix 169

Carnival on Ice...170

Carob Classic 170

Chai Green...171

Cherie's Green Morning Blend..................................171

Chia Mia 172

Chocolate Chimps..173

Cocoa Cabana 173

Coconut Creamsicle...174

Simple fun with Green Smoothie.............................174

Smoothie of Aloe Vera...175

Smoothie of Skin...176

Smoothie of Aloe 177

Strawberry Fun..177

Lemonade with Aloe Vera 178

Superfood Smoothie 179

Mean Green Smoothie 180

Basil Smoothie with Strawberry 181

Basil Berry Smoothie 182

Awesome fun with Aloe Vera 183

Cilantro of Tropical Smoothie..................................184

Smoothie of Cilantro Recipe 185

Fruity Green Smoothie...185

Green Coconut Smoothie...187

Banana Avocado Green Smoothie............................188

Green Milk Smoothies 189

Spinach Yogurt Smoothie 191

Green Lime Pie Smoothie 192

Tropical Green Blast Smoothie 193

Caramel Banana Green Smoothie 194

Mango Spinach Green Smoothie..............................196

Zucchini Vanilla Green Smoothie.............................197

No-Fruit Green Smoothie...199

Pineapple and Coconut Spinach Smoothie................................200

Nice Lettuce Punch Smoothie..201

Lovely and Sour Green Smoothie 202

Green Smoothie Bowl with Mango + Hemp Seeds...................204

Snickerdoodle Green Smoothie 205

Green Warrior Protein Smoothie 206

VEGAN MANGO-COCONUT GREEN SMOOTHIE 208

Low-Carb Shamrock Protein Smoothie 209

Tropical Green Smoothie 210

Blueberry & Peanut Butter Green Smoothie 212

Metabolism Boosting Green Smoothie 213

Scrub Yourself Clean Green Smoothie......................................214

Purple Passion Green Smoothie 216

Strawberry Banana Green Smoothie 216

Apple Pie Green Smoothie 217

Electric Green Boost...218

Sweetie Pie Green Smoothie 219

Mango Cucumber Green Smoothie..220

Green Tropical Sunrise 221

Kale Almond Milk Smoothie...222

Introduction

The name "Green Smoothie" says is all!

Green smoothies are those smoothies that are made with green vegetables & fruits. You cannot make use of food color in a green smoothie. They may be better than the standard smoothies with regards to taste, nutrition value, and whatnot. That's the reason this book is focused on green smoothies.

Green smoothies are well ... green! Maybe not green in color, although some of these are, however they are green in contents. They might be fruit blended with a few of nature's additional magical ingredients. Some are light and fresh and tangy. Others are smooth, luxuriant, sweet, and creamy. Others have a citrus note, others taste more herb-laden.

Whatever your targets, whether it's your search for vibrant health, weight reduction, or shape management, incorporating green smoothies would be the revelation you have already been searching for!

There is no greater gift compared to the gift of great health.

Taking this positive step may be the way to bring yourself back and in ways where you can have the results within you as well as the clarity in your thoughts.

With the present-day age of processed food items, there are more prepared foods and only pre-packaged food and less of the focus on fresh produce. With so many enticements to go from the types of foods, we ought to be consuming one really must be careful never to stray too much through the (garden?) path.

When you assume control and begin pumping in the nice nutrients that processed stuff becomes much less attractive. You're likely to discover your cravings will morph, your shopping habits right along with them. Vegetables and fruits are believed as the utmost healthy food on the planet. This is the major reason behind saying green smoothie as the very best smoothie. Going for a green smoothie is better than ingesting salad having a dish. You can find the reasons for this. The main reason is usually, you can eat a whole lot of greens whenever you have a smoothie.

It isn't possible to consider a lot of healthy ingredients with salad. So, Smoothie is your best option. *Green smoothies won't cause you fat related problems.* These are wise and healthy. You will not be suffering from stomach related problems regardless of just how much you consider green smoothies and they're wonderful against heart-related diseases. You will discover individuals who will let you know that green smoothies usually do not taste as effective as the standard smoothies. Yes, this is true to an extent but there are several options for you to choose from. Unless you like one smoothie then do not waste your time and effort there. Simply proceed to another one which is guaranteed that you'll like at least a number of the recipes if not absolutely all out of this book. Green smoothies are filled with minerals and vitamins. It'll satisfy your hunger plus the nourishment level at the same time.

Chapter 1

What are Green Smoothies?

To be able to maintain a sound body, we have to guarantee we look after the body. This includes a healthy diet plan, followed by a dynamic lifestyle as well as choosing standard health checkups and caring for any issues that arise before they turn into a problem. A very important factor that lots of people often argue about is usually breakfast while one band of individuals claim breakfast to become the main meal of your day, additional groups have a tendency to argue against the fact and declare that breakfast may only contribute to an unhealthy weight. The simple truth is, breakfast can be an important part of life. It's the initial meal of your day as well as the meal that will get you during the day by providing the body with nutrients that may support high energy and fight off any signs of fatigue.

We explain a healthy breakfast can provide a person with benefits, such as improved concentration throughout the day, better mental and physical performance as well as the strength that's needed to partake in activities. It will contribute towards a nutrient-rich diet that supplies your body with vitamins for skincare, mental care also to contribute to the overall wellbeing of the body. Besides, they explain a healthy breakfast has shown to keep up lower degrees of cholesterol throughout the entire day.

What are Green Smoothies

Today we will take a look at how drinking a green smoothie for breakfast time might help improve your current wellbeing.

To begin with, a green smoothie is, as the name suggests, green in color. This green color is gained from all the green fruits & vegetables that are put into these smoothies. Simple Green Smoothies explain a green smoothie is manufactured out of green leafy vegetables, coupled with nutrient-rich fruits and finished with a liquid base. Besides, they explain that lots of people choose to top their smoothies off with some superfood.

Daily Life Improvements Caused by Green Smoothies as Breakfast

With all the current goodness of spinach, broccoli, kale, and several other leafy greens, coupled with some deliciously tasty fruit, green smoothies for breakfast might help you make some healthy changes in your daily life.

Increases Your Daily Fruit & Vegetable Intake

We live busy lives that a lot more than often causes us to just forget about how crucial fruits & vegetables are throughout the day. Whenever we are busy, we tend to grab the nearest snack when hunger strikes, and these snacks usually will not be a healthy choice. By starting your entire day having a green smoothie, you already are consuming a whole lot of vegetables & fruits, thus boosting your regular intake of the essential food types. Not merely will this contribute to your current health, but you will soon learn how to improve memory through adequate daily nutrition.

SFGate reports that the common active individual should consume as much as three cups of vegetables regularly, as well as around two cups of fruit. Green smoothies tend to include a massive amount both fruit and veggies, therefore you won't need to be worried about your day-by-day intake just as much as you will often have to.

Promotes weight reduction Naturally

Green smoothies are abundant with many minerals and vitamins that support the human body's general health, but they may also be a fantastic addition to a weight reduction regimen.

Improves Hydration

Water can be an essential daily substance that people need. Our anatomies are mostly made up of water, and we have to keep our anatomies hydrated to aid our health and wellness. The average individual must consume around 2.7 liters of water each day this does take into account water intake that people gain from beverages and foods. Unfortunately, many folks are not happy using the taste of water. Simply by adding more water to your green breakfast smoothie, you can consume yet another amount of liquid, which increases the 2.7 liters you will need to consume day-by-day.

Improves Digestion

Just as much as 70 million folks are suffering from some digestive disorder. These disorders could be due to numerous factors, including an *inactive lifestyle and an unhealthy diet*. Green smoothies are filled up with fiber, which is a superb substance to greatly help improve digestion and could offer relief towards the symptoms which are due to common digestion disorders.

Rejuvenates the body

The things that are contained in green smoothies contain chlorophyll. It has benefits for your body and besides features powerful antioxidant properties. Organic Facts explain that chlorophyll can prevent anemia, help with dental problems, reduce symptoms of sinusitis as well as support treatment of insomnia. Apart from this, chlorophyll improves the disease fighting capability and may rejuvenate the complete human body.

Protects Against Free Radical Damage

In addition to the chlorophyll content material (which can be an antioxidant), green leafy vegetables also contain a great many other antioxidant. Antioxidants have many health advantages. Probably one of the most common benefits of antioxidants may be the fact that these compounds can protect our body from free radical damage, which is a term used to spell it out unstable molecules within your body's cells.

Reliefs Symptoms of Depression

The high concentrations of folic acid that are located in green leafy vegetables are recognized to support the relief of the signs of depression. Reports also state that folks who have problems with depression frequently have a folic acid (or folate) deficiency.

Better, & Clearer Skin

We often spend a huge selection of dollars every month on skincare products. your skin is in the end, the very first thing someone sees if they first meet you. Green smoothies are saturated in vitamin E and vitamin C, as well as fiber and antioxidants. Many of these chemicals work together to give you an improved complexion and clearer skin - without costing a lot of money.

It is an acknowledged fact that it is better we look after our anatomies, the healthier we have been, this means we won't need to face the results of the unhealthy lifestyle regularly. This, however, appears to be a hard task for many individuals. We would introduce you to green smoothies. These delicious smoothies will also be filled with nutrients and make a fantastic breakfast. They provide a vast selection of health benefits that may help you get through your day, as well as support your future wellbeing.

Chapter 2

Green Smoothie Health Advantages

Green Smoothie health advantages among absolute favorite self-care activities are usually to start every day by using a freshly blended green smoothie!

They are a good way to get five or even more servings of fruits & vegetables every day.

Green smoothies were instrumental in weight loss. Drinking a green smoothie each day, will reduce your cholesterol level, your energy will fly through the roof, and your skin stays healthy,and radiant shine.

Below are a Few of the Very Best Health Advantages of Green Smoothies:

Natural fat loss

Just about everybody who drinks green smoothies loses weight. Green smoothies assist you to lose weight in several ways:

First, replacing meals each day which has a green smoothie lowers overall calorie consumption, while increasing fruit, vegetable, and fiber intake.

Secondly, green smoothies help reset your tastebuds so you want to consume healthily, and you truly start craving well-balanced meals.

Boost Fruit & Vegetable Intake (Particularly Greens)

The American Cancer Society recommends that people eat 5-9 servings of vegetables & fruits each day to avoid cancer along with other diseases. Green smoothies certainly are a quick and convenient way to get your vegetables and dark, leafy greens without tasting them.

The fruit masks the flavor so even though whatever you taste is pineapple, mango, banana, or strawberry, you are consuming a wholesome dose of spinach, kale, or any other vegetable which you put in.

The common green smoothie contains 3-5 servings (or even more) of fruits & vegetables.

Increased Energy

Green smoothies give a powerful boost of vitamins, minerals, antioxidants as well as other nutrients without bogging down your digestive tract. Because you are eating natural, whole foods within the most optimum kind for the digestion and nutrient absorption, you should have more vigor to get things done and revel in your day.

Green smoothies provide B vitamins and magnesium that help support energy metabolism.

Boosts Nutrition

Green smoothies are jam-packed filled with nutrients.

The common green smoothie recipe provides a lot more than 100% of the day-by-day value of vitamins A (as beta-carotene), C, and K. Also, they provide a sound way to obtain B vitamins (except B12), vitamin E, and folate.

As for nutrients, green smoothies are loaded with calcium, iron, magnesium, manganese, phosphorus, potassium, copper, and several other trace minerals.

Blending vegetables & fruits together reduces the cells of plants and improves digestibility. Your blender unlocks the nutrients and maximizes their delivery to the body a lot more than chewing any salad could.

Green smoothies are quicker and far more convenient than preparing and thoroughly chewing a salad.

Strengthens disease fighting capability (Immunity)

Increased fruit and vegetable consumption helps maintain the body in optimum health. Vitamins, minerals, and antioxidants, as well as a number of the compounds within certain foods, support to protect the body against disease. Citric fruits, cranberries, and ginger will be the top immune-boosting smoothie ingredients.

Got a sniffle? Make an effort these cold and flu green smoothie recipes!

An excellent way to obtain Minerals For Healthy Bones

Green smoothies give a rich way to obtain minerals because of the dark, leafy greens. All the bone-building nutrients are abundant including calcium, magnesium, and phosphorus. A lot of my green smoothie recipes in this book contain much more than 200 milligrams of calcium, and several have significantly more calcium when compared to a glass of milk.

Excellent Way to obtain Antioxidants

Green smoothies deliver an enormous dose of health-protecting antioxidants and phytonutrients. Not merely are you currently giving the body the very best defenses against disease, you are ingesting several natural substances that are crucial for optimum health.

To obtain the most antioxidants within your mixes, try making your green smoothies with blueberries, strawberries, cranberries, pomegranates, acai, and cacao (raw chocolate).

Can help Lower raised cholesterol

A wholesome, plant-based diet which includes green smoothies can help decrease your cholesterol.

Can help Lower High blood pressure

Many fruits & vegetables have already been studied for its capability to lower blood pressure.

Within a healthy diet plan, green smoothies may increase your blood pressure, while also reducing the number of the risk factors for coronary disease.

Improves Mental Clarity and Focus

With a wholesome diet comes greater mental clarity and focus. Green smoothies have replaced my morning coffee ritual.

I get more strength from a green smoothie, and there isn't any afternoon slump or caffeine-related unwanted effects.

Supports Colon and Gut Health

Unlike juicing or drinking the juice, green smoothies support the entire fruit and vegetable so you get every one of the fiber and nutrition.

Fiber is vital once and for all colon health. It feeds your beneficial gut microbes, supporting optimum digestion and a solid immune system.

Promotes Crystal clear, Radiant Skin and Strong Hair & Nails

Lots of people say that their skin, hair, and nails look healthier and stronger while drinking green smoothies. It has certainly been my experience. Green smoothies give me a wholesome glow, plus they solved my adult acne.

Reduces and Combats Cravings

Green smoothies reduce cravings for junk food, unhealthy sweets, salt, and fats. You will see that after a couple of weeks of drinking smoothies, you may crave healthier foods such as fruits, vegetables, and greens.

The sweet fruit in green smoothies satisfies cravings for sweets. If you crave chocolate, you may make green smoothies with healthy, raw chocolate (cacao).

Anti-Inflammatory

Most vegetables & fruits have anti-inflammatory properties, so green smoothies are fantastic food if you have problems with inflammatory conditions.

A lot of people report that drinking green smoothies each day reduces inflammation.

Green Smoothies can help Prevent Chronic Diseases, as well as Provide Therapeutic Benefits

There were countless studies on diet and nutrition. The overwhelming consensus in every from the peer-reviewed, scientific literature is definitely that folks who eat even more fruits & vegetables have a lesser threat of developing the disease - including cancer, diabetes (type-2), obesity, coronary disease, as much as age-related medical ailments. *Specifically, green smoothies, coupled with healthy diets, might provide therapeutic benefits for (or drive back):*

✓ ***Supports Eye Health & Protects Vision:*** Green

smoothies are abundant with beta-carotene, lutein, zeaxanthin, and resveratrol antioxidant compounds within many vegetables & fruits.

✓ ***Specific Benefits for ladies:*** Certain fruits & vegetables, and also other smoothie ingredients, can help women who have problems with PMS. Women going right through menopause could also reap the benefits of green smoothies.

✓ ***Can help with Seasonal Allergies:*** As the medical data is bound, there are numerous, many reports of individuals who've reduced the severe nature of the seasonal allergies after they started drinking green smoothies.

✓ ***Rich with Chlorophyll:*** Green smoothies are rich with chlorophyll which some natural health experts say enhances the disease fighting capability, purifies the blood, and rejuvenates your body.

While these claims tend over-hyped, it doesn't hurt to get potentially beneficial plant compounds in what you eat. If you do desire to increase your consumption of chlorophyll, then obtain it from leafy greens and miss the questionable supplements.

- *__Alkalizing:__* Many natural health experts promote the alkalizing effects of green smoothies (or vegetables & fruits). This claim is controversial, however. Promoters in the acid-alkaline "theory" declare that green smoothies help neutralize blood pH and stop your body from becoming too acidic. The simple truth is that no food causes blood pH to improve, therefore green smoothies could not affect neutralizing blood pH as your body tightly regulates it (using whatever you take in). Green smoothies provide minerals that can be used by the body to naturally maintain pH balance. The calcium, magnesium, and phosphorus in leafy greens help maintain your bones strong. If you're not deficient, the body doesn't have to rob your skeleton of the precious minerals.

  Also, a lot of people have pointed out that heartburn and indigestion disappear when drinking green smoothies.

Furthermore to these health advantages, green smoothies are:

- Easy to create and tidy up after.
- Taste amazing.
- Will make any couple days in the refrigerator.
- Are fun to create and test out different fruit and vegetable combinations.
- Green smoothies are life-changing!

Chapter 3

Green Smoothies

Many experts think that a wholesome lifestyle starts with an excellent breakfast. Research demonstrates you will find significant benefits for individuals who *"rise and dine,"* such as:

- A diet that's more nutritionally complete and higher in nutrients, minerals, and vitamins,
- Improved concentration and mental performance,
- Even more physical strength and endurance,
- Lower cholesterol levels,
- Offers a metabolic boost that assists with weight reduction,

Yet with all this research and overwhelming evidence showing the need for eating a wholesome breakfast, only 1 third of adults who want to eat breakfast, do eat it. Everybody knows at fault behind missing breakfast-lack of your time.

There's a solution. One which is simple and quick to prepare, affordable, and most crucial -healthy!

Green Smoothies

Green smoothies act like traditional fruit smoothies but contain much more green veggies and include *spinach, lettuce, kale, collard greens, parsley, dandelion greens, watercress leafy green veggies your palate desires. Bananas, apples, pears, avocado, and mango* are excellent companions for these kinds of smoothies and work very well to improve the entire flavor and texture.

Chlorophyll Rich

Green smoothies are rich with chlorophyll which some natural health experts say enhances the disease fighting capability, purifies the blood, and rejuvenates your body. It is among the multiple reasons why these delicious drinks are touted by experts to be loaded with energy for the body.

Helps to improve mental clarity and focus

Leafy vegetables are filled with antioxidants and carotenoids, which increase your brainpower and help protect the human brain. Also, they are filled with B-vitamins, that are proven to support your memory, focus, and overall brain health insurance and function. Also, they are abundant with folic acid, which improves mental clarity.

It's never easy to remain healthy using a busy schedule. That is why you will need a program to remain motivated to do this goal.

Assists with digestion and overall metabolic function

Unlike fruit drinks, green smoothies utilize the whole fruits & vegetables so you get all the fiber and nutrition. Fiber is essential for all colon health insurance and it keeps your bowels in working order. These smoothies naturally combat constipation and help promote regularity.

Blending vegetables & fruits together reduces the cells of plants which improves digestibility. The blending action unlocks the nutrients and maximizes their delivery to the body much better than chewing a salad could. Smoothies are a competent and far more convenient way to benefit from every of the health benefits, in comparison with preparing and eating a salad, especially on the run.

Increases consumption of fruits & vegetables

The American Cancer Association recommends that people eat 5-9 servings of vegetables & fruits each day to avoid cancer along with other diseases. Green smoothies certainly are a quick and convenient way to get your vegetables and dark leafy greens without tasting them. The fruit masks the flavor, so even though whatever you taste may be the fruit, you maintain consuming a wholesome dose of spinach, kale, carrots, and some other vegetable you add.

Improves mood and helps fight depression

Green veggies contain plenty of folic acids which is a natural antidepressant. The folate within greens helps fight memory loss and increases serotonin levels, which results in improved moods.

Promotes natural weight loss

Green smoothies are filled with nutrition and so are surprisingly low in calories. They support the vitamins, minerals, healthy carbohydrates, fiber, and zero fat entire food you'll want to lose weight promptly, safely, and effectively without starving yourself. Also, they are lower in sugars found naturally in fruit and fruit drinks, making them a wholesome option than traditional fruit smoothies and natural juices.

Clearer skin

Clearer, radiant skin can be an often-reported benefit to eating healthier. Smoothies are saturated in fiber and invite your body to remove toxins correctly rather than through your skin layer. The vitamin E within green leafy vegetables works with vitamin C to help keep skin healthy while you age.

Hydration

Drinking green smoothies isn't just a terrific way to trick yourself into eating your vegetables, additionally, it is an effective way to make sure you get the water the body needs. One of many factors many people usually do not drink the recommended 6 to 8 glasses of water daily is because they simply do not like the taste of plain water. If that describes you, add more water to the mix when you ready your smoothie. You will be drinking more liquids without even noticing it.

Green smoothies certainly are a wonderful breakfast alternative. You may receive all the benefits of consuming breakfast while simultaneously reaping the advantages of ingesting your veggies.

Is Your Green Smoothie Vibrant?

Green smoothies are the hype nowadays, but there's much confusion about how to obtain the most out of this day-by-day dose of feel-good medicine.

Among the chief reasons you'd want to swap your dead, sugar-laden, complex breakfast having a "pre-chewed" living greens smoothie is to get the use of bioavailable nourishment while preserving your precious digestive system. In this manner, the body can focus its energy on other important tasks, like cellular repair, detoxification as well as the metabolism of this not-so-healthy late-night snack.

Unlike popular belief, it's not essential to start your engine completely force as soon as you awaken. Possess your lemon water, take your probiotics, vitamin D, iron, and B12, then get blending.

Add more greens

If you'd like your smoothie to become healthy, keep carefully the *alkalizing greens dominant (60-80%).* Understand that these greens shouldn't ever compromise the taste. *Have them in, mask them with some low to medium GI fruit, and some delicious supplements, and both your belly as well as your palette remain satisfied.*

Easy, neutral-tasting greens include romaine and spinach. Focus on these and you'll get hooked. Other fun greens to try out with consist of kale, collard greens (stems removed), butter/red/green lettuce, fennel, celery, cucumber, and herbs (cilantro, mint, and parsley - in smaller quantities).

If you're overwhelmed from the taste of pungent or bitter greens, halve the total amount and substitute with romaine or spinach.

Use low glycemic fruit

A spike in blood sugar levels is not essential for anybody, no matter what time. Because that's usually accompanied by an accident, and we certainly don't want to feel just like we need a nap at 11 o'clock each day. To maintain your blood sugar balanced, nearly all your fruit ought to be low GI, using a smaller level of medium-labeled fruit. ***Low GI fruits*** *include apples, pears, grapefruit, kiwi, oranges, strawberries, and plums, while* ***medium GI fruits*** *include bananas, mangoes, papaya, and pineapple, to mention a few.*

When you can, adhere to organic varieties. If this isn't possible, shop from your Clean 15 - you'll be surprised just how many delicious fruits and vegetables produce the cut!

You must be aware that everybody will react differently to food combinations and health claims. The main element is to test out yourself, cautiously, and openly. I put in a ripe banana to my daily smoothie and also have never experienced an accident or felt poor at all (bloating, gas, headache). Others may beg to differ. I say adhere to low GI, play with the medium GI options, and pay attention to your body.

Make use of supplements! But make certain they're clean

Nowadays, it's not enough to trust our fruits & vegetables alone to supply us with adequate nutrition. Not because they're not amazing for your wellbeing, but instead it is due to the grade of the soil where these were grown their way to obtain health. When the soil is deficient, to begin with, just how do we expect our whole foods to surpass our expectations?

That's where organic and local also enter into play. If we just choose organic, often those varieties must travel the world to access our kitchens. Much like globe-trotting humans, the procedure of air/ship/land distribution is tiresome, energy-depleting, and potentially toxic.

So, back again to supplements. These babies are nutritious, specific, delicious (some, anyway), and accessible. Some supplements could also enhance the absorption of nutrients from your living foods into the gut, making them essential to obtaining that spare umph out of the day-by-day smoothie. I'll offer my suggestions predicated on the desired health advantages themselves and appearance out for multi-functional duplicates!

Listed below are my top supplement suggestions, with some key, but nonexclusive benefits noted:

Fiber: chia seeds (soluble and insoluble), flax seeds, psyllium husks

Protein: spirulina, chlorella, nuts (almonds, walnuts, brazil nuts), seeds (sunflower, pumpkin, sesame, chia, flax, hemp) - or their respective butter, mesquite, lucuma, carob

Minerals and vitamins: maca (B12, iron, calcium, libido boost), lucuma (potassium, magnesium, phosphorus), ashwagandha (antioxidant, adaptogen, ideal for men), Shatavari (calcium, zinc, excellent for women), cacao (antioxidants, magnesium), carob (potassium, calcium), mesquite (calcium, magnesium, potassium), matcha green tea extract (antioxidant)

Healthy fat: coconut (meat, oil, butter), avocado, nuts (almonds, walnuts, brazil nuts), seeds (sunflower, pumpkin, sesame, chia, flax, hemp - the latter which offers both omega-3 and -6).

Low GI sweet tooth satisfiers: stevia leaf powder or extract, Medjool dates, lucuma (naturally sweet), mesquite (nice, caramelly flavor), coconut nectar

Miscellaneous healers: vanilla bean powder, cinnamon (blood sugar levels regulator), ginger (digestive), turmeric (anti-inflammatory), cayenne (gut cleaner)

Switch it up frequently and mindfully

This one is true for some things in life. Performing a similar thing, again and again, will get boring and overwhelming, physically, emotionally, and regarding health, internally. There's a substantial amount of discussing dark leafy greens like spinach and chard containing oxalates, which block or reduce calcium absorption, but this shouldn't quit anyone from using these greens unless indicated professionally.

Diversity also pertains to fruits and supplements. If you've been adding an apple for your smoothie this week, make use of a pear in a few days. Bring flax today and hemp tomorrow. On days whenever your lovely tooth dominates, toss in some surplus lucuma or mesquite. Maybe a good pinch of stevia or perhaps a date or two. Replace your drinking water base with coconut normal water or even homemade nut milk. For the daring or for all those trying to avoid a cold, utilize a tea base, like immune-boosting chaga or reishi.

Switch it up, make smoothie prep fun and you'll observe how promptly it becomes an integral part of your routine.

My final tips and thoughts:

Blend your greens first and add the rest of the ingredients and blend again. This creates more room for other goodies. If you're addicted to blending, consider buying the almighty **Vitamix**. It'll turn your smoothies into pure decadence. Other high-speed blenders are the **_Blendtec and Nutribullet_**.

If you'd prefer to creamify your smoothies, put in a little bit of whole-food healthy fats, like avocado (1/2 is enough), coconut meat (2 tbsp), or a small number of nuts or seeds (nut butter, seed butter, and milk included).

Don't forget that digestion begins in the mouth area! Activate those salivary enzymes by "chewing" your smoothie. If you draw unnecessary attention from bystanders, simply embrace and welcome it - unless it's warranted from your green mustache!

Chapter 4

Immune Boosting Smoothies for Breakfast

Good, the greens in each smoothie support the minerals and vitamins the body needs for hormonal balance. The fiber through the greens also feeds the microbiome within your gut, which means that you absorb these minerals and vitamins. Finally, protein helps calm your hunger hormones, letting you possess a four- to the six-hour window of satiety without feeling as if you have to snack before the next nutrient-dense meal.

Make an effort one or most of my immune-boosting smoothies! These low-sugar recipes certainly are a nice, satisfying way to start your day.

Squeeze in a few lemons

My go-to Spa Smoothie includes avocado, spinach, mint leaves, and a refreshing touch of lemon. Continue steadily to reap immune-boosting great things about lemon during the day with the addition of a slice to some cup of tepid to warm water each day, or squeeze lemon juice on your salad when eating out.

Spa Smoothie

Ingredients

- ✓ 1 scoop vanilla protein powder
- ✓ 1/4 avocado
- ✓ one to two 2 tbsp. chia seeds
- ✓ juice of just one 1 lemon
- ✓ couple of spinach (fresh or frozen)
- ✓ 1 small Persian cucumber
- ✓ 1/4 cup fresh mint leaves
- ✓ 2 cups unsweetened nut milk

Directions:

Place all ingredients inside a high-speed blender and blend to the required consistency. If you are using frozen spinach, there's you don't need to bring ice. If you are using fresh spinach, you can include a small couple of ice to cool the smoothie.

Pro Tip:

The oils within the mint leaves can help rehydrate you naturally when you feel beneath the weather. Steep some peppermint tea and store it inside the refrigerator, then use it rather than nut milk as the bottom of your respective smoothie for an invigorating kick!

Pack in those greens

This simple but delicious kale smoothie is chock-full of leafy greens containing vitamins A and C, fiber, and calcium. The beta carotene in kale also delivers a youthful glow by increasing pigment within the skin and potentially neutralizing free radicals. Almonds will also be a great way to obtain antioxidants and nutrients.

Ingredients

- ✓ 1 serving Primal Kitchen Vanilla Coconut Collagen Protein
- ✓ 1 tbsp. almond butter
- ✓ 2 tbsp. flax meal
- ✓ couple of kale
- ✓ 1 cup unsweetened almond milk

Directions:

Place all ingredients within a high-speed blender, and blend to the required consistency. If you want to cool it down, put in a small couple of ice.

Acai Green

Delicious blueberries and acai contain vitamin C! Besides, they contain **anthocyanins**. They are plant anti-oxidants from the capability to lower cholesterol levels, fight oxidative stress, and assist in preventing aging.

Filled with vitamin A and fiber, the acai fruit is a skin superhero. The spinach with this smoothie can be a great way to obtain omega-3s, potassium, calcium, iron, magnesium, and vitamin B, C, and E.

Ingredients:

- ✓ 1 serving organic vanilla pea protein
- ✓ 1/4 - 1/2 avocado
- ✓ 1 tbsp. chia seeds
- ✓ couple of spinach
- ✓ 1 tbsp. acai powder
- ✓ 1/4 cup organic frozen or fresh wild blueberries
- ✓ 2 cups unsweetened almond milk

Directions:

Place all ingredients inside a high-speed blender, and blend to the required consistency. If you aren't using frozen blueberries, you can include a small couple of ice to cool it down.

Coconut Turmeric Cream

Turmeric contains medicinal properties called *curcuminoids*, the main of which is usually curcumin. Curcumin may be the ultimate "anti." It's been proven to demonstrate antioxidant, anti-inflammatory, antiviral, antibacterial, antifungal, and anticancer activities.

Another key element of this smoothie is its *medium-chain triglycerides (MCT)*. MCTs certainly are a healthy fat that may reduce inflammation by killing off bad bacteria, such as candida or yeast, that may overgrow inside our intestines. They're also known for increasing energy, decreasing weight, and supporting appetite control. MCTs frequently result from coconuts. They're a definite, tasteless oil that's easy to increase smoothies.

Put in a few raspberries to the smoothie to up your intake of vitamins A, C, and E!

Ingredients:
- ✓ 1 serving Primal Kitchen Vanilla Coconut Collagen Protein

- ✓ 1 tbsp. coconut butter or MCT oil
- ✓ 2 tbsp. Now Foods Acacia Fiber
- ✓ 1 cup unsweetened almond milk
- ✓ 1 tbsp. Goldyn Shine Turmeric Maca Powder (Energy Blend)
- ✓ 1/4 cup frozen or fresh raspberries

Directions:

Place all ingredients within a high-speed blender, and blend to the required consistency. If you aren't using frozen raspberries, you can include a small couple of ice to cool it down.

How does these smoothies boost the immune system?

Spring feels as though it ought to be, but we're technically even now in the center of cold and flu season. During this period of the entire year, I love to support my clients get a supplementary immunity boost with vitamin C.

Vitamin C plays an integral role inside the disease fighting capability: It stimulates the production of white blood cells, that assist fight infections. It could also decrease the timeframe contamination stays in the torso.

The Smoothie formula of protein, fat, fiber, and greens is guaranteed to nourish the body with what it requires to carefully turn down hunger hormones, keep you satisfied all night, and limit excessive sugar. They're also a good way to improve your consumption of vitamin C, as they're plentiful in leafy greens, citric fruits, berries, as well as an avocado!

Chapter 5

History of The Green Smoothie

Green smoothies are well-liked by those seeking a wholesome lifestyle.

Touted as the perfect healthy snack and a good nutritious meal replacement, green smoothies are located on many café and street vendor menus. Their rise to fame is related to the increased popularity of medical and weight-loss shakes which have swept the country. Consumers looking for a far more nutrient-rich, dairy-free or low-fat option, helped to create the green smoothie towards the forefront. With fresh, organic produce easily available, more folks are embracing the green trend, whipping up green smoothies in the home. Believers within the green smoothie are reaping medical great things about these fresh satisfying concoctions which are void of preservatives and additives. The thing is the green smoothie is not a fresh sensation.

Traditionally, a smoothie is a blended drink, manufactured from fruit, milk, and yogurt.

Some recipes demand fruit juices to avoid milk products. Over time this blend is becoming more specialized and today features many variations. *It's important to indicate that smoothies aren't milkshakes. Smoothies use whole fruits & vegetables, whereas milkshake will bring flavor enhancers and sweeteners to milk. Smoothies are usually thicker when compared to a milkshake too. Smoothies aren't only created from the juice of vegetables & fruits either; therefore their vitamins and minerals do differ compared to that of juicing foods.*

That is an important differentiation, normally juicing is performed to take pleasure from the flavor of sure fruits & vegetables. With regards to green smoothies, the vegetables aren't always selected for his or her taste. Their essential vitamins, minerals, and soluble fiber far outweigh any flavor they increase a drink.

Who coined the brand *"smoothie"* is not known. The oldest patent from the title belongs to Stephen Kuhnau, who established the 1970s Smoothie King franchise. But historically, the idea of a smoothie traces backward further. The original drink of India referred to as a "lasse" bears an extraordinary resemblance to some smoothie. It is a mixture of yoghurt, fruit, honey, and spices, and was around b.c Christ. In Brazil, drinks manufactured from fruit purée blended with yogurt also feature in antiquity.

Strangely enough, thick, creamy drinks containing avocado along with other fruits are traditional fare in Vietnam, the Philippines, and Indonesia. The 1920s and 1930s saw entrepreneurs promote these foreign elixirs in health stores over the West Coast of America.

As technology developed, so did the smoothie. The 1920s saw the birth of household appliances. Homes shortly filled up with machines that made life easier. Among these highly valued kitchen accessories was the blender. The 1933 "Miracle Mixer" is accredited because of its efforts in establishing the "smoothie" as the children's name. Combined with the improved models released well into the 1940s, all featured smoothie recipes within their accompanying cookbooks. As the technology developed machines with the capacity of combining ingredients into smooth, thick liquids, the smoothie became popular.

From the 1960s, typical smoothie blends saw fruits, fruit drinks, or milk being whipped together in tasty treats. The 1970s embraced the trend of using frozen yoghurt in smoothies. The 1980s added supplements; tinkering with protein and vitamin powders. Yet it had been the 1990s that heralded a fresh smoothie renaissance, having a baby into a multi-billion dollar industry.

Victoria Boutenko introduced the green smoothie at the same time when smoothies are more popular than ever before. Sick and tired of constant, niggling medical issues, *Boutenko decided to make an effort the all-natural, raw foods diet*. Within the 1990s, she subjected herself, and her family, to ten years long diet that strictly had them eating meals abundant with green, leafy produce.

Strangely enough, her research compared the typical American Diet with the normal diet in our closest living relative, the chimpanzee.

She discovered that chimps ate a diet plan of at least forty percent leafy greens and 50 percent fruit. The highly promoted raw-food diet encouraged extremely high levels of fruit and recommended only 10 % of leafy greens each day. Boutenko began exploring the advantages of increasing the greens within their diet. Predicated on her research, and her own family's experiences, *Boutenko found green smoothies to become the best health choice.*

Victoria Boutenko recommended that the average individual needed to consume at least four servings of green leaves or more to four pounds of fruit every day. Although a lot of people could stomach the fruit, munching down large portions of salad leaves became a chore. *Further research also revealed that the entire vitamins and minerals of green leafy vegetables were only fully gained once the cell walls in the leaves were chewed, or cut.*

The smaller the leaves are shredded, the better these were for the digestive tract. This information resulted in the introduction of the green smoothie. With a high-grade blender, green leafy matter such as spinach was very easily chopped right into a smooth substance that mixed perfectly with fruit and just a little water. The generous serving of fruits masked any bitter taste of several fresh leaves, creating glass or two that was highly nutritional; so the green smoothie revolution began.

Today, many folks are experiencing great things about drinking green smoothies. You will find a huge selection of recipe books and websites that focus on creating varied and tasty versions of the health tonic. Green smoothies promise to provide a low-calorie, highly nutritional boost to the dietary plan. They contain essential vitamins and trace elements that may only exist sourced from your hero with the drink, the green leafy vegetables. Green smoothies are thought to assist with digestive issues but are also recommended to help ease arthritis rheumatoid and several allergies as well as other health issues. Today, the green smoothie is constantly on the evolve as fresh mixes and products are explored.

Tips to make Green Smoothies

healthy smoothies require a base for creaminess, some liquid, then your fruit and/or veggies, plus added ingredients for extra nutrition.

For the bottom, most greens along with other smoothie makers use either banana, avocado, and/or mango or papaya to make them creamy. For various other fruit smoothies, you should use yogurt for any creamy texture as well as for spare bulk and diet you can include oats to any smoothie. Alternately, nuts make an excellent base because they are extremely creamy once you blend them with some water.

Bananas are excellent if they are ripe. Then they possess a few black and brown spots to them and are filled with minerals and vitamins. They contain fiber, vitamin A, C, E, K, thiamine, riboflavin, niacin, B6, folate, B12, and pantothenic acid. A banana will put in a sweeter taste for your smoothie and hide most of the green taste. It could also solidify after one hour and also you could offer a green smoothie dessert!

To create green smoothies palatable for kids, add more banana, mango, or frozen berries-the the sweetness could keep the greens hidden.

For different fruit smoothies, you should use yogurt, cream, or creme fraiche to get a creamy texture. Some individuals prefer never to make use of dairy for health reasons and I have chosen to go dairy-free for weight loss so that as a healthier decision but please do your research upon this subject matter. For surplus bulk and nourishment you can even contribute oats to any smoothie.

If you wish to avoid fruit, then avocados provide a thick texture to some smoothie and offer vital nutrients and phytochemicals-just get them to ripe (not black and dented).

A view on avocados and fat content

They contain all 18 essential proteins and thus certainly are a complete protein that's simple to digest. Besides, they contain "healthy fat" which improves the so-called "sound" cholesterol, which helps drive back free radical damage and diabetes. They can be abundant with carotenoids (for eye health) and so are anti-inflammatory. *The primary fat in avocados is oleic acid, which is proven to improve heart health.*

Besides they contain many omega-3 essential fatty acids, which are recognized to lower the threat of heart disease. System that you might worry about is the great sort of fat! If you're starting a healthy diet plan, attempting to lose weight, or going "raw," one or two avocados each day can help you create the transition because they will fill you up and limit your cravings. My advice is to simply pay attention to your body. While you get healthier you might need less or prefer less good fat in what you eat or may very well not. Limit your bad fat intake or cease altogether. It is possible to adjust the quantity of avocado you utilize within a green smoothie according to your needs-less if you're just using a snack smoothie, even more, if you work with it as a meal replacement. I like the taste of avocado in my smoothies but unless you, then reduce the amount to 25% of the avocado and supply considerably more banana or mango.

Using mango and/or pineapple and coconut milk together will provide you with a tropical taste to any smoothie.

For any boost for the nutritional value of the smoothie, you can include *wheatgrass powder, whey, or other protein powders, maca, flax seeds, or other green powders like spirulina.* Just adding among these will put more "vigor" to the smoothie, so experience a few handy.

You can test other liquids within your smoothie apart from cow's milk and water.

Almond milk, hemp milk, juiced veggies or fruit, and coconut milk as suggested above, will all put in a different taste and consistency.

Green smoothie enthusiasts will venture out trying to find green leaves in gardens themselves and pick edible leaves and blend them up. You truly do need to know what's edible and what not to do. I might advise you never to do this if you are not 110% certain of everything you are picking, as some leaves are poisonous. adhere to what you will get locally from markets and shops and look out for in-season produce to improve up your regular.

There will never be any recipes with this book with hard-to-find ingredients!

Other ingredients to get handy are *honey, maple syrup, the sugar substitute xylitol, or the sweet herb stevia.* Nevertheless, you should just need these if you're not using much fruit nevertheless, you want just a little sweetness for your smoothie. *The juice of carrot, beetroot, pomegranate, or extra berries or banana should offer you enough sweetness without resorting to sweeteners.*

Suggested Superfoods

superfood is a term to spell out foods that can be densely filled with nutrients and really should be contained in your daily diet. I often utilize a ready-made powder made up of something similar to green barley grass or wheatgrass.

However, if you're juicing and blending plenty of vegetables and fruit every day you ought not actually to need extra superfood powder. Having said that, many people might need a supplementary boost. It is also handy if you're out of green veggies or simply want to create something fruity but put in a little "green."

There's a huge set of foods given that are usually known as "super," but below are a few you could easily find you need to include in a smoothie:

Blueberries

Saturated in fiber and antioxidants, blueberries certainly are a top superfood.

Blue-green algae

Will come in powder form and maybe the richest way to obtain chlorophyll that you can buy. It is a substance that cleans your blood and detoxifies. Also, an excellent way to obtain protein, beta-carotene, and B12.

Brazil nuts

A terrific way to get a great dose of selenium, zinc, protein, magnesium, and thiamine. You can throw several these into the blender once in a while and they'll smooth out good. I've seen it recommended you don't eat even more than one or two 2 brazil nuts per day for their high selenium content; they can become toxic in high doses, and besides, increase your LDL cholesterol.

Cacao

Raw chocolate, an exceptionally rich antioxidant, and filled with iron, magnesium, and chromium as well. It is stated to improve your mood, lower cholesterol, and enhance the circulation of the blood. Cacao also includes phenethylamine that is reported to produce greater focus and cause you to even be more alert. The phytochemicals in cacao are reported to be an aphrodisiac. Remember it can contain some caffeine as well. You may get raw cacao nibs or powder in your neighborhood health store. Can make your smoothie chocolatey!

Coconut

Good for strength, losing fat, and is an excellent way to obtain fiber, iron, and manganese. Additionally, it is reported to boost your thyroid function.

Guava

That is packed filled with vitamin C, plus fiber, potassium, manganese, and folic acid.

Maca

Also known as *Incan superfood*, it's been utilized for a large number of years by Andean societies to nourish and heal. Benefits include increased stamina, endurance, and libido, which is also thought to stimulate tired adrenals and the complete endocrine system to revive vitality. It includes amino acids, nutrients, vitamins, alkaloids, and sterols (ideal for bodybuilders!). It includes a vanilla/caramel taste and is fantastic in smoothies.

Mesquite Powder

Some individuals put this within their smoothies. It is ground in the pods inside the mesquite plant and continues to be eaten for a large number of years by Native Americans. *It is abundant with protein, fiber, potassium, iron, zinc, calcium, and lysine, and it is very proficient at balancing blood sugar levels as the sugar within it is fructose and will not require insulin to metabolize it.*

As a side note, *if you're diabetic or hypoglycemic, green smoothies might help your condition.* You could stick to simply veggies, tomato, and avocado, no fruit or surprisingly low sugar fruit, and add milled flaxseed, flaxseed oil, or hemp seed oil in your smoothies, which helps decelerate the digestion and release of sugars.

Pomegranate

Filled with antioxidants as well along with the seeds contain fiber. *Its benefits include the prevention of blood clots, reported to be always a natural cure for prostate cancer, can prevent heart disease, reduces diarrhea, reduces plaque in arteries, lowers blood circulation pressure, and so many more.*

Raspberries

Saturated in fiber, antioxidants, as well as other nutrients.

Spirulina

This is a kind of blue-green algae and an excellent way to obtain protein, EFA's, minerals, and vitamins. The iron is effective for all those with anemia. It is stated to greatly help with fat loss, detoxify the body, improve blood glucose problems, remove toxic metals from your body, and lower cholesterol, among other benefits.

Wheatgrass

This is best for chlorophyll, enzymes, proteins, minerals, and vitamins.

Benefits include increasing red blood cell count, reducing blood pressure, assisting to detoxify your body, neutralizing poisons, and alkalizing your body. It'll strengthen your cells, it is thought to restore fertility, turn gray hair on track color, as well as freshen your breath!

This is only a short set of the countless superfoods accessible to you. In case you check out your neighborhood health grocery you'll be certain to get assorted superfoods in powder kind that may provide your smoothie with this increased nutrient boost.

Should You Buy or Make Your Milk?

Adding milk is a superb option for your smoothies. It can help produce a creamier and thicker consistency than simply adding water. So go on and happily then add organic cow's milk, goat milk, hemp seed milk, or almond milk to the next creation.

Cow's milk has come under scrutiny recently with some medical researchers now saying it's harmful to us in support of baby cows ought to drink it!

However, some doctors say that organic raw milk is okay to drink since it is usually unpasteurized as well as the healthy bacteria and enzymes remain intact no artificial HGH can be found. Goat's milk is reported to be much healthier.

When you get almonds, get the nice variety which has been pasteurized, instead of raw almonds-these certainly are a safer choice.

You should use brazil nut milk in moderation-as aforementioned, brazil nuts could be toxic in large doses.

Hemp seeds are excellent for protein because they contain eight proteins and they are a "complete" protein. They include a high amount of omega-3 essential fatty acids, vitamins, and minerals.

Pumpkin seeds also make excellent milk.

How to make your milk

You'll find oat, nut, and seed milk in the store, but if you want to create your own, then utilize this procedure:

✓ Soak your nuts overnight before blending. (Hemp seeds don't need soaking; just rinse). Rinse the soaked seeds or nuts.

- ✓ Have a cup of the selection of seeds or nuts.
- ✓ Devote a blender and add 3 to 4 cups of filtered or clear water.
- ✓ Add a couple of dates or just a little honey, xylitol, stevia, agave nectar, or cinnamon and also a little vanilla, extract-these are optional based on your taste.
- ✓ Blend and pour via a sieve or strainer as well as for better still straining, subjected to a cheesecloth.
- ✓ This will provide you with thick milk.
- ✓ To get a thinner consistency, add more water in the initial mix or blend using the strained milk.
- ✓ Refrigerate and store as normal milk but shake before employ in case there is separation.

Chapter 6

Set of Fat-Burning Foods and using Smoothies for Weight Loss

Certainly, you can slim down by drinking green smoothies! Substitute your regular snacks of cookies, poker chips, or additional unhealthy foods having a smoothie for an excellent beginning to healthy eating and weight loss.

The best thing about smoothies is the fact that once you begin drinking them you will observe that you will not feel so hungry for unhealthy snacks, your time can last longer, and it'll become even better to scale back on breakfast or lunch. You will likely be equipped for a good dinner though-make convinced it's healthy!

To accelerate your fat lose, make an effort to add fat burning foods within your smoothies-check out the list following:

Apples

They are filled with a dietary fiber called pectin that assists you in feeling fuller for longer.

Apples also contain Vitamin C. Apricots Abundant with fiber, apricots assist you to experience fuller longer and can help lower blood cholesterol levels. They include a large amount of beta-carotene, which helps mop up free radicals and increase your immune system.

Beets

Beets certainly are a natural diuretic; this means they'll help get rid of excess water weight or fluid. They have got iron, fiber, and natural chlorine, which can only help rinse toxins and fats out of the body. Due to the iron content in beets, they certainly are a wonderful food for those who have anemia.

Broccoli

Broccoli is filled with fiber as well, and abundant with vitamin C, which may dilute system.drawing.bitmap and helps it be easier to remove from your own body. Contains vitamin B, calcium, iron, beta-carotene, and may help lower blood circulation pressure and detox your liver. Only use several florets per smoothie since it is fairly bitter tasting-you can juice it first and add it for extra "green."

Blackberries

Full of fiber, vitamin C, along with other nutrients.

Blueberries are believed a great belly fat fighter. They may be filled with phytonutrients, antioxidants, and so are low-calorie if you're being careful.

They certainly are a low-sugar fruit, so they certainly are a wise decision if you're sensitive to sugar.

Cabbage

Sulfur and iodine in cabbage help cleanse your intestines and stomach. Cabbage also includes calcium and vitamin C.

Cantaloupe

Best for vitamin A and C, potassium, vitamin B6, soluble fiber, folate, and niacin (vitamin B3), and fiber.

Carrots

Make an extremely sweet juice to increase smoothies, they may be saturated in vitamin A and so are an excellent detoxifier, and support your liver and guts function smoothly.

Celery

This can eliminate skin tightening and from your system and its pure type of calcium will feed your urinary tract.

Hormones out of this part of your body assist to split up fats. Contains magnesium and iron and it is an all-natural diuretic.

Cherries

Take away the stone before blending! These are supposed to decrease pain and inflammation and contain anthocyanin that is said to give rise to stomach fat reduction.

Chives

Support with weight loss because of the high chromium content. *Chromium* is a nutrient that improves the functioning of insulin within the bloodstream.

The even more stable your insulin, the greater stable your blood sugar and the considerably more stable your time is, resulting in fewer cravings!

Cranberries

Lower in sugar, plus ideal for the urinary and digestive system. Ideal for fighting cellulite and detoxifying the body.

Cucumbers

An excellent fat-burner because like a diuretic, they'll encourage removing waste fluids from your own body. There are also good levels of silica and sulfur to stimulate the kidneys to flush out the crystals in the torso. Best for nails, skin, and hair, and will reduce blood circulation pressure.

Dandelion greens

Dandelion leaves and roots are accustomed to treat various ailments and boost health by Europeans, Asians, and Native Americans. The greens stimulate the liver, kidneys, and digestion, and become a diuretic.

Goji berries

Fantastic for antioxidants and contain protein, essential minerals, and proteins. You can purchase these dried. Ideal for blood building as well as the immune system.

Grape fruit

Grapefruit can help your body's insulin amounts to contribute to a fat-loss regime.

Green beans

Lower in calories, abundant with nutrients. Improve liver, kidney, and lung functions.

Green beans have vitamin C and iron, which both fight fat.

Honeydew melon

Great for dietary fiber as well as for high water content, so will increase your hydration on the hot daytime, plus deliver minerals and vitamins to the body.

Juniper berries

Help eliminate excess fluid retention and improve digestion. Also, they are anti-inflammatory! Never to be consumed by women that are pregnant or women desperate to conceive as juniper could cause uterine contractions.

Kale

Kale is an associate of the same family as Brussel sprouts and broccoli. High in fiber possesses many nutrients, so excellent for dieters.

Lettuce

Full of minerals and vitamins and best for your metabolism with thermogenic properties. (Thermo Orange genic fruits and vegetables are lower in calories but need a lot of vigor to digest, thus raising your metabolism once you eat them, which can help you burn up more fat.)

Lemons

A squeeze of lemon is ideal for wearing down fat and cleansing your body.

Limes

Filled with fat-fighting vitamin C!

Mango

Filled with fiber but lower in calories, an excellent way to obtain beta-carotene and vitamin C.

Nectarine

Has protein, fiber, and is filled with nutrients. The calcium, magnesium, and potassium promote fluid balance, so these are best for weight loss.

Oatmeal

Adding some oatmeal to some smoothie might help you drop weight since it is saturated in fiber, which can only help stabilize your blood sugar levels, and that means you are less inclined to snack on unhealthy snacks.

Orange

Ideal for their high vitamin C content and fiber.

Papaya

Papaya is fat-free possesses fibers, A, C, potassium, calcium, iron, thiamine, riboflavin, and niacin. Also includes the enzyme pepsin, which helps dissolve fat in the torso. Please buy organic as papaya is usually genetically modified.

Peaches

Packed with nutrients and vitamins and fiber. They can be full of fiber content, making them filling.

Pears

Contain a high fiber quite happy with vitamin C and calcium.

Pineapple

Pineapples support the enzyme bromelain, which helps digest protein and can be anti-inflammatory. Also, they are a great source of fiber, thiamine, vitamin B6, copper, vitamin c, and manganese.

Pumpkin seeds

Also known as pepitas, they are delicious crunchy snacks that are abundant with manganese, tryptophan, magnesium, and phosphorus. They are usually anti-inflammatory agents as well.

Raspberries

The raspberry is a good fat buster due to its high fiber content and low sugar level. The pectin in raspberries can help prevent an excessive amount of fat from being absorbed into the cells, thus helping fat loss.

Spinach

Filled with iron, it'll increase your metabolism when consumed regularly and can promote better liver function.

Strawberries

Filled with powerful antioxidants, and they also lessen inflammation and increase metabolism. Might help control blood sugar.

Tomato

Sound vitamin C content plus contains phytochemicals that produce carnitine. Carnitine helps to breakdown fat within your body so that it can be utilized for energy.

Watermelon

Contains plenty of dietary fiber and mineral deposits and is ideal for your metabolism.

Watermelons will hydrate you because of their high water content making them ideal for smoothies.

Other Fruits and Vegetables and their Vitamins and Minerals

Avocado

My favorite decision in green smoothies, they can be saturated in protein, potassium, fiber, many vitamins including A, E, C, B6, and K, and healthy unsaturated fats for sustained energy.

Bananas

Contain vitamins, nutrients, and antioxidants. Particularly known for it high fiber, high potassium, vitamin C, and B6 content. Ideal for a quick strength boost because of the simple sugars content.

Coconut

Beneficial in smoothies as water or milk. Packed with antioxidant, it helps your body numerous functions including digestion, cell building, sugar amounts, weight-loss, and metabolism-and it's antibacterial too. It includes a higher concentration of electrolytes than some other food. So excellent for hydration!

Dates

Contain many minerals and vitamins, particularly saturated in fiber, iron, potassium, and antioxidant beta-carotene.

Fennel

Best for fiber, vitamins, and antioxidants.

Ginger

Anti-inflammatory and antibacterial. Helps reduce nausea, migraines, and diarrhea (due to e. Coli). It includes nutrients including vitamins B5 and B6, potassium, magnesium, and manganese.

Grapes

Abundant with resveratrol, which is a powerful antioxidant, however, they are quite sweet, so be cautious when you have a sugar problem.

Passion fruit

A very good way to obtain antioxidants, fiber, vitamins, and nutrients, particularly vitamins C, A, and potassium.

Prunes

Very abundant with vitamin A and antioxidants. Full of dietary fiber and ideal for constipation!

Kiwi

Great way to obtain vitamin C and E, potassium, and folic acid. Best for blood pressure, heart health, disease fighting capability health, and digestion. Can help you find rest from blockage and bloating.

Red cabbage

Plenty of vitamin C as well as other minerals and vitamins plus fiber.

Nice bell peppers

Rich way to obtain minerals and vitamins particularly vitamin C in debt pepper and everything contains high vitamin A content. Capsaicin can be an alkaloid within these peppers, that is reported to be best for cholesterol levels and can be anti-bacterial, and anticarcinogenic, with benefits for diabetics.

Other Green Smoothie Greens

Collard greens

A good way to obtain phytonutrients which have anti-cancer properties. Ideal for vitamins A, K, and C and different minerals.

Mustard greens

High in vitamin K, and best for vitamins A and C, and also a higher level of folates and fiber.

Rocket or arugula lettuce

Abundant with phytochemicals that fight assorted cancers such as breast, prostate, and ovarian. Provides minerals, particularly calcium and iron plus vitamin K and vitamin C.

Romaine lettuce

Very abundant with vitamin A, plus folates, vitamin C and K, B vitamins, and iron.

Swiss chard leaves

A rich way to obtain vitamins A, C, and K plus iron and omega-3 essential fatty acids. If regularly used, it is stated to greatly help iron-deficient anemia, prevent osteoporosis and different heart diseases plus some cancers.

Turnip greens

Has high degrees of antioxidants, vitamins A, C, E, calcium, and copper and is also reported to be useful for all those with arthritis.

Watercress

Ideal for vitamin A, C, and K, betacarotene, and different minerals. You will see a great many other green veggies inside the supermarkets such as spring greens, bok choy, etc. Feel free to experiment!

Chapter 7

Choosing Your Greens

Here's what you ought to do:

1. Taste what's accessible to you

2. See whether it's mild, medium or strong in its taste and,

3. Vary your consumption. Remember never to take just a few types of greens.

4. Have several inside your refrigerator every week. Change from week to week and that means you can buy quite a lot of state, 4 types instead of smaller amounts of articulate 8 varieties.

Storage and Use for Smoothies

In my mind, it's better to have everything No problem finding and use. I would recommend washing, drying, and storing your greens so that they're accessible at a moment's notice. You want everything to be as effortless as possible. That will continue steadily to inspire you to help expand success and much more vibrant health. It'll keep you on the right track to make sound decisions too (instead of reaching for the 'wrong' stuff!).

Below you'll discover some suggestions. If you like different ways then opt for that.

TIP: *Wash your greens once you get home!*

I believe you will need to make yourself up for success! I've found an invaluable move to make is to clean your greens whenever you bring them a house (or in from your garden). Fill your kitchen sink so the leaves you might have afloat.

Take away the twist ties or elastic bands or other packaging from your greens.

Take off the roots of plants that you don't need or plan to employ. Separate whatever leaves need separating through the stem. Clean the dirt off. Look for little bugs because they are doing hide within especially if you get organic produce.

Other Essentials

Various other essentials certainly are a blender, an excellent knife, and a chopping board. Consider various other items that could motivate you including juicers, books, ebooks, a particular knife, or possibly some fresh glassware for the smoothies.

Smallest amount: You will need recipes, knife, blender as well as your produce.

Drying Your Greens

Make use of a colander to strain a lot of the water from your leaves. If that is what you did and put them within the refrigerator your greens would still perish. Drying them is vital. So drain them and move them in the colander into a clean dry tea towel which you layout over a bench, table, or in a bowl. You can pat the leaves dry. When you have a very useful salad spinner.

While it could be frustrating, it's worth the time and effort to spend enough time to process your greens immediately. It truly is a pleasure to really get your washed and dried greens from the refrigerator and pop them directly into the blender.

Storing Your Greens

Place the greens into bags or boxes. When you do, place the tea towel or some kitchen paper which to sit your greens so that condensation is mopped up plus the greens have less connection with the plastic (that may cause some spoiling).

Stems

You don't have to discard the stems. Many recipes will tell you firmly to only utilize the coriander leaves (cilantro). With green smoothies, you can use extra of the plant. Appreciate using even more of your parsley, coriander as well as mint. Simply stay away from the woody stems as thick and fibrous green stems won't blend well.

Some people think that the stems possess the least nutrition. This isn't the situation. However, they have more fibers and so could be less enjoyable in salads. The upside is usually they are loaded with flavor and fiber to your smoothies.

Why Green Foods?

Green foods have become likely probably the most nutritionally precise foods to meet up the needs of humans. Let's go through the ways they will be the perfect food to nourish every cell, prevent risk, and keep us lean and energetic.

Protein

Let's start with protein since people under western culture are rather preoccupied with this topic. Certainly, protein (along with carbohydrates and fats) is necessary inside our diet which is, indeed, very vital that you build up muscle mass and keep maintaining the fitness of tissues through the entire body.

Folks are consistently shocked to discover that, for example, broccoli and spinach are a lot more than 40 percent protein. But protein content material is only a great way that greens are often the ideal, nourishing, disease-preventing foods anywhere in the world.

If you're seeking to increase protein within your plant foods for a particular health reason, consider that spinach is highest, at 42% protein, and utilize it liberally inside your green smoothies (while also obtaining a selection of greens). Make an effort to produce your smoothies as lower in fruit as easy for your taste, and consider making the no-fruit smoothie.

You can simply add protein powder, though most whey- and soy-based protein powders are fractionated, heat-treated, rather than healthy. Many studies before decade show that soy isn't medical food we thought it was for quite some time. Soy in its whole and fermented forms, found in moderation, tend entirely appropriate. The issue is that we're being bombarded with too much soy using prepared isolates (elements of the grain separated from the complete food). Soy lecithin, soy proteins, and several different derivatives are in a large number of supermarket offerings. Please avoid soy protein powders.

Chlorophyll and blood-building properties

Among the factors greens are powerhouse foods may be the plant energy produced from chlorophyll, which may be the plant exact carbon copy of hemoglobin inside the human red blood cell. Chlorophyll neutralizes internal body odors and bad breath, and it mops up free radicals that cause cancer and everything degenerative disease.

Calcium

Everyone understands that calcium (coupled with vitamin D obtained by spending a moderate timeframe in sunlight) builds strong bones. Many people believe that milk products are their finest resources of calcium. While dairy is saturated in calcium, it's not particularly bioavailable to humans. The foodstuffs highest in calcium highly useable by folks are, obviously, greens. Highest are collards, parsley, watercress, dandelion greens, beet greens, kale, and watercress.

Unequaled nutritional profile

Greens certainly are a powerhouse of enzymes, vitamins, and nutrients. They may be, ounce for ounce, probably the most nutritionally dense foods on earth because they're the lowest in calories and highest in micronutrients. Scientists have recently discovered several nutritional classes of micronutrient compounds, but we nonetheless don't understand how they all interact to safeguard against cancer and disease. What we do know is the fact that greens, unlike synthetic vitamins, contain those compounds that synergistically reduce our threat of myriad health issues.

Most leafy greens are saturated in antioxidant vitamins A, C, and E that bind with and neutralize free radicals. They're a way to obtain folic acid that aids in preventing birth problems in babies, as well as magnesium, which can be an easy nutrient to be deficient in. Their dark colors show that they're saturated in phytochemicals, including over 500 carotenoid antioxidants, flavonoids, and indoles working synergistically to provide the eater of greens abundant health. No supplement can offer an ideal balance of nutrition that raw green food contains naturally.

Fiber

An incredible number of Americans rely on chemical derivative fiber supplements to pay for his or her low-fiber diet. (Chemical drinks like Metamucil won't be the same as natural plant fiber and may irritate and overstimulate your body's digestive tract.) That is a tragedy with epic consequences, not least which is usually skyrocketing cancer of the colon deaths. The colon is going to be healthy if we offer it, the whole day, with plenty of insoluble plant fiber. That bulk drags the space in our gastrointestinal tract, much just like a broom, keeping its tissues clean and pink and healthy.

Fibre famously prevents all sorts of cancers and digestive problems, but it additionally reduces cholesterol and cardiovascular disease and controls blood sugar levels by slowing sugar uptake within the bloodstream. It prevents gallstones, decreases diabetes risk, binds excess estrogen, and assists in weight loss by creating a feeling of fullness and less wish to overeat.

You don't find many foods higher in dietary fiber than greens. The insoluble fibers function such as a sponge inside the gut and will expand, absorb, and remove many times its weight in toxic materials. Its importance can't be overstated because it's the only path we must move dead cells and several additional wastes through your body in minimal time, preventing the decomposing and diseased cells that result when food sits, undigested, in a variety of elements of our digestive and elimination systems.

A quart or even more green smoothie day-by-day is a phenomenal way to dramatically increase fiber in the dietary plan. A quart should provide 12-15 grams of fiber to your daily diet. The common American gets only 11 grams of fiber daily, so if you're from the standard American diet, your fiber will at least double with the addition of this single habit. The USRDA is 30 grams, though government standards are rather unambitious, politically motivated, lowest common- denominator standards. You truly need 50-70 grams. Don't be daunted by those figures. Make a gradual increase but, most importantly, don't stay at the normal American's 10-15 grams each day, where your disease risk is quite high.

Way to Save Money on Green Smoothie

After people overcome the original hurdle of wondering just what a green smoothie tastes like and learning it can be quite nice, their next objection may be the cost. "Those ingredients are costly!" they state, or, "Just how much does a blender filled with that stuff cost?!"

Generally, before offering my cost-saving tips, I wish to explain that eating plenty of raw greens can prevent a lot of health problems which you truly can't afford never to eat them. You'll surely save over time whenever you aren't coping with the expensive unwanted effects of illness, obesity, as well as a large number of attendant risks of the normal American lifestyle.

That said, listed below are ten ideas to save money-the the first two could have an enormous cost-saving effect on your finances if you're ready to invest a little bit of cash and time up-front. The payoff of implementing simply the very best two ideas with this list can be quite rewarding.

Figure out how to Garden

With just a little planning, you could have almost-free, organic green smoothie ingredients year-round. Grow a garden that has greens prominently.

Figure out how to garden through the wintertime, and freeze the excess greens within the warm growing season. Spinach, chard, and kale have become simple to grow in backyard or patio gardens, and by the end of the summertime, you can replant for any fall harvest that explodes again inside the spring through the frost season. Chard, specifically, produces an enormous amount of green food and will not bolt easily in warm weather; by staggering plantings, I harvest it from a couple of weeks following the spring frost until well following the last fall frost. Also consider that carrots, beets, turnips, radishes, and strawberries now provide a fresh food source for you as the green elements of those plants you might have been throwing out before are ideal for your smoothies.

Choose Large Freezer

This is the second-highest-important idea to those who find themselves frugal or strapped for cash: Choose a large freezer.

Harvest Edible Weeds

Several greens could be harvested from vacant lots in town when the elements are warm. Edible weeds within most climates include lambsquarter leaves, nettles, morning glory, and purslane (as well as thistle).

Purslane includes a very mild flavor and texture for addition to smoothies; it's an unusually rich way to obtain omega-3s and iron. Be sure you do not use weeds you aren't sure are edible.

Dandelion weeds can often be bitter but are plentiful generally in most climates, and I often throw a few within the blender. Avoid picking these weeds in areas next to busy roadways, as greens absorb the toxins in car exhaust fumes. Also, avoid any areas which have been sprayed with pesticides or weed killer. Dandelion greens are least bitter if they are picked inside the spring before they bloom with yellow flowers.

Buy in Bulk

Bananas, pears, frozen strawberries, and frozen mixed berries will also be significantly less expensive frequently at some supermarket than in a few other food markets.

Shop at Health Food Stores

Monitor the contents of medical food stores locally. Within my local health grocery, although organic bunches of kale, collards, and chard are admittedly more costly than conventional produce, the bunches are much bigger, therefore the higher price is typically not higher per ounce. In cases like this, paying more is warranted to get more reasons than simply nutrition.

Freeze fruit

Buy fruit for sale and in season, and freeze it before it goes bad. if you start to see the bananas are getting black and can't utilize them all, peel them, break them into chunks, and put them in sandwich baggies within the freezer. you can purchase a lug or two of peaches when they're in season, and wash and quarter them in baggies to freeze and last through the wintertime.

Freeze Fresh Greens

Greens, too, while they can't be frozen for salads along with other purposes, could be easily frozen for later make use of in smoothies. Nobody can tell. And that means you do not have to allow spinach to go south again.

Buy Frozen Spinach

You can purchase frozen spinach in the wintertime when fresh spinach is quite expensive, and occasionally those boxes or bags of spinach inside the freezer section are less costly.

Support Local Growers

Discover the community-supported agriculture and health-food-buying co-op groups locally. They'll have money-saving deals on organic produce that may bring your costs down.

Be familiar with small markets locally

Get familiar with the market near your house which has excellent prices on interesting greens like various cabbages (yu choy, bok choy, tatsoi, and several others), as well as fresh ginger, several vegetables, and young Thai coconuts.

Chapter 8

Greengrocery

Traditional Greens/Lettuces

- ✓ Kale
- ✓ Red chard
- ✓ Butter lettuce
- ✓ Miner's lettuce
- ✓ Arugula
- ✓ Spinach
- ✓ Napa cabbage
- ✓ Tatsoi
- ✓ Parsley
- ✓ Rainbow Swiss chard
- ✓ Endive
- ✓ Romaine
- ✓ Mache
- ✓ Vegetable amaranth
- ✓ Red cabbage
- ✓ Bok choy
- ✓ Pac Choi
- ✓ Radicchio
- ✓ Swiss chard

- ✓ Escarole
- ✓ Mixed greens (mesclun)
- ✓ Celery
- ✓ Collard greens
- ✓ Green cabbage
- ✓ Yu Choy
- ✓ Mizuna

Tops of root vegetables

- ✓ Beet greens
- ✓ Turnip greens
- ✓ Grape leaves
- ✓ Kohlrabi tops
- ✓ Carrot tops
- ✓ Dandelion greens
- ✓ Mustard greens
- ✓ Jerusalem artichoke tops
- ✓ Strawberry tops (organic)
- ✓ Radish greens
- ✓ Anise/Fennel greens

Sea Vegetables

- ✓ Arame
- ✓ Nori
- ✓ Kelp
- ✓ Kombu
- ✓ Hijiki
- ✓ Wakame
- ✓ Dulse

Weeds

- ✓ Purslane
- ✓ Lambsquarter
- ✓ Morning glory
- ✓ Japanese knotweed
- ✓ Creeping Charlie

Sprouts

- ✓ Brocolli sprouts
- ✓ Fenugreek
- ✓ Quinoa
- ✓ Bean sprouts
- ✓ Radish
- ✓ Pea greens
- ✓ Alfalfa

✓ Clover

Herbs

✓ Mint leaves

✓ Lemongrass

✓ Bay leaves

✓ Tarragon leaves

✓ Marjoram

✓ Cilantro (coriander)

✓ Basil leaves

✓ Horseradish root

✓ Chives

✓ Oregano leaves

Fruits for Green Smoothies

They are ingredients you may consider, which list is in no way comprehensive.

✓ Apricots

✓ Apples

✓ Bananas

✓ Blackberries

✓ Blueberries

- ✓ Boysenberry es
- ✓ Cherries, Bing
- ✓ Cantaloupe
- ✓ Cherries, pie
- ✓ Cranberries
- ✓ Crenshaw melon
- ✓ Grapes
- ✓ Guanabana
- ✓ Grapefruit
- ✓ Honeydew melon
- ✓ Kiwi
- ✓ Kumquats
- ✓ Lemons
- ✓ Limes
- ✓ Marionberries
- ✓ Mango
- ✓ Nectarines
- ✓ Oranges
- ✓ Papaya
- ✓ Pears
- ✓ Peaches
- ✓ Persimmons
- ✓ Pineapple

- ✓ Plums
- ✓ Prunes
- ✓ Raspberries
- ✓ Star fruit
- ✓ Strawberries
- ✓ Tangerines
- ✓ Tangelos
- ✓ Watermelon

Kale - Abundant with folate, vitamin C and K, calcium, iron, and beta-carotene. It's also a hormone balancer, digestion booster, anti-inflammatory, possesses omega-3 essential fatty acids.

Grapefruit - Abundant with vitamin C and is a superb detoxifier for the liver.

Cucumber - Prevents fluid retention, promotes a wholesome digestive tract, filled with bioavailable nutrients, vitamins, and electrolytes.

Celery - Abundant with fiber and B vitamins, prevents fluid retention

Apple - Way to obtain fiber and vitamin C, helps balance blood sugar, boosts digestion, reduces inflammation

Algae oil (DHA rich) - A sustainable, plant-based way to obtain omega-3 essential fatty acids. My go-to brand is NutraVege. Creating 97% of the fatty acids present in the mind, DHA is an essential long-chain fatty acid within the omega-3 family. It's super very important to women that are pregnant and children beneath the age of 2 since it supports brain, vision, and nerve development. Note: I don't add this oil straight into the smoothie. I just consider it separately so that it doesn't impact the flavor.

Virgin Coconut Oil - Coconut oil has antiviral, antifungal, and antibacterial properties. It's abundant with medium-chain triglycerides (MCTs) that assist raise the metabolism and lower the chance of cardiovascular disease.

Hulled hemp seeds - An excellent way to obtain complete protein, provides the best balance of omega 3-6-9 essential fatty acids, and is saturated in fiber. Hemp seeds also reduce inflammation in the torso and balance hormones.

Mango - Abundant with vitamin C, fiber, and beta-carotene. Besides, it contains enzymes that assist with the break down of protein in the torso (ideal for the above mentioned protein-rich hemp seeds.

Chapter 9

Green Smoothies Recipes

Cashew Blast

- ✓ 5-7 Kernels of Cashew Nuts
- ✓ Spinach Leaves
- ✓ Lemon Syrup
- ✓ Curd
- ✓ Sugar

<u>Directions</u>

Half boil the spinach leaves and remove its raw appeal. Mix the lemon syrup and thick curd thoroughly inside a bowl. Grind cashew kernels and sugar to provide a coarse mixture. Place the half-boiled leaves into the curd and bring the coarse cashew kernels with sugar. Finally, blend just a little to provide a uniform texture. Enjoy this smoothie with bread toasts.

Yogurt with Cinnamon

- ✓ 1 Ripe Cucumber
- ✓ 1 cup Oat Milk
- ✓ A pinch of Cinnamon
- ✓ Salt

- ✓ Coriander Leaves
- ✓ Probiotic yogurt

Directions

Chop the cucumber into mid-sized pieces and blend all ingredients except cinnamon within a grinder. Place it into the refrigerator for some time. Right before serving, put in a pinch of cinnamon and garnish with coriander leaves.

Peanuts with Mint and Honey

- ✓ Peanuts without shells
- ✓ 1 handful Mint Leaves
- ✓ Thick curd
- ✓ Honey
- ✓ Ice cubes

Directions

Grind all ingredients together to create a thick uniform paste. Lastly, add the ice and serve cold.

Kiwi Guava Burst

- ✓ 1 Kiwi

- ✓ 1 Guava
- ✓ Coconut Water
- ✓ Fresh Corn Kernels
- ✓ Ice Cubes

Directions

Chop the kiwi and guava into small pieces. Grind the corn kernels with coconut water and add the chopped fruit pieces involved with it. Serve with ice.

Spinach Surprise

- ✓ Bread Slices
- ✓ Spinach Leaves
- ✓ Yogurt
- ✓ Lemon Syrup

Directions

Blend the spinach leaves in yogurt. Add bread slices and blend again to obtain a thick texture. Add lemon syrup to taste and serve at room temperature.

Lychee with Eggs and Honey

- ✓ Egg whites
- ✓ Milk
- ✓ 7-8 lychees
- ✓ 2 cucumbers
- ✓ Honey

Directions

Blend the egg white thoroughly with milk and honey. Peel and chop lychees into small pieces and keep aside. Blend the cucumbers using the milk mixture. Add the lychee pieces in a way that they float within the smoothie. This gives flavor and taste like none other.

Almond and Banana

- ✓ 1 Medium Banana
- ✓ Cubed Pineapple Pieces
- ✓ Fresh Mint Leaves
- ✓ Roasted Almonds
- ✓ Ice Cubes

Directions

Cut the almonds into fine pieces and keep aside. Blend the banana, pineapple and mint leaves as well as ice to provide slush like mixture. Garnish with sliced almonds right before serving.

Lettuce with Yogurt and Orange

- ✓ Organic Lettuce Leaves
- ✓ Fresh Thick Yogurt
- ✓ Orange Pulp
- ✓ Ice

Directions

Blend the yogurt with orange pulp to provide a smooth pulpy texture. Half boil the lettuce and add the chopped leaves into the yogurt mixture. Blend thoroughly. Finally, add crushed ice to the mixture and serve chilled.

Pear and Banana Blast

- ✓ 1 Organic Pear
- ✓ Coriander Stalks
- ✓ Milk
- ✓ 1 Ripe Banana
- ✓ Sugar

Directions

Chop the pear into smaller pieces and keep aside. Crush the coriander stalks in milk. Add the ripe banana to milk and blend well. Add sugar to taste and add the chopped pear pieces towards the smoothie. As a choice, you can include mint leaves into the smoothie to improve the taste and flavor.

Banana Berry Smoothie

Ingredients:

- ✓ Spinach- 2 cups
- ✓ Banana- 1 piece
- ✓ Mixed berries0 3/4th cup
- ✓ Raw nuts- ¼th cup
- ✓ Water- 1-2 cups

Directions:

1. Make certain the banana is ripe. It ought to be peeled too.

2. You can even usage strawberries or blueberries in it. Choose sunflower seeds or flax seeds for the raw seed category.

3. You can even use coconut drinking water unless you want to utilize the normal one.

4. Now to put it simply everything inside the blender and switch it on. Blend it for just two minutes. Enjoy.

Strawberry with Lemonade

Ingredients:

- ✓ Kiwi - 1 piece
- ✓ Fresh strawberry- 3/4th cup
- ✓ ¼ - ½ cup pineapple
- ✓ Lemon- ½ cup
- ✓ Spinach- 2 Cups
- ✓ Normal water- 1.5 cup

Directions:

1. You should use coconut normal water instead of standard drinking water if you'd like. The lemon must be peeled.

2. The kiwi also needs to exist peeled. Now put everything around the blender and switch it on.

3. Blend it for just two . 5 minutes. Remove it. Enjoy.

The Glowing Smoothie

Ingredients:

Organic lettuce- 1 piece

1.5 cup of water

Organic spinach - ½ head

Apple- 1 piece

Pear- 1 piece

Banana- 1 piece

Lemon juice- ½ tbsp.

Directions:

1. Simply put normal water in a blender. Another task is usually to put spinach in it. The secret here is to start slow and increase.

2. Begin the blender at minimal speed and slowly raise the speed and mix it till it gets smooth.

3. If you are increasing the speed, slowly add everything involved with it. Bring the lemon juice by the end.

4. It ought to be done within five minutes. Enjoy.

Fight to become Well Smoothie

Ingredients:

Kale- 3 stalks

Lettuce - 3 leaves

Coconut drinking water- 1 cup

Banana- 1 piece

Blueberries

Hemp Seeds- 1 tsp

Chia Seeds- 1 tsp

Bee Pollen- 1 tsp

Maca Powder- 1 tsp

Spirulina- 1 tsp

Directions:

1. The producing Direction isn't tough because of this recipe. To put it simply everything within your blender simultaneously.

2. Then switch it on and make the smoothie. That's it. Enjoy.

Powder of Green Smoothie

Ingredients:

Oat Milk- 1 cup

Coconut Drinking water- 1 cup

Spirulina- 1 tsp

Flaxseed meal- 2 tsp

Coconut oil- 1 tbsp

Berries- 1/4th cup

Probiotics- 1tsp

Organic yoghurt- 2 tbsp

Cinnamon

Stevie- 2 drops

Directions:

1. Turn your blender on. Ensure that the coconut oil that you will be using is organic. Also, yoghurt needs to be organic.

2. You ought not to use a lot of cinnamon. Just a pinch will be adequate.

3. To put it simply everything within the blender and transform it on.

4. Blend it for three minutes and serve. Enjoy

Renewal Smoothie

Ingredients:

Spinach- 1 bunch

Mint- 1 handful

Parsley- 1 handful

Lemon juice- 1tbsp.

Lettuce Leaves

Stalks- 4 celery

Cucumber- 1 piece

Ginger- 1 piece

Ice- 5 cubes

Directions:

1. Ensure that the spinach is English as well as the ginger can be peeled properly.

Turn the motor on and pour everything onto it.

2. Usually do not put ice inside the blender. You must put ice at the top of the smoothie to obtain a cool feeling.

3. Make an effort to sip it slowly to get an extra taste. Enjoy.

Greeny Green- Beginner's Luck

Ingredients:

Spinach- 2 cup

Normal water- 2 Cup

Mango- 1 piece

Pineapple- 1 Cup

Banana- 2 piece

Directions:

1. The process is simple. Make certain the spinach is certainly fresh and tightly packed.

2. Now turn the blender on and juice it for at least three minutes.

3. Use ice to create it cool. Enjoy.

Cilantro with Mango Detox

Ingredients:

Spinach- ½ cup

Cilantro- ½ cup

Mango- ½ cup

Drinking water- 2 cups

Pineapple- 1 cup

Avocado- ½

Directions:

1. It is a straightforward one to produce. The first thing you'll want to do would be to blend the spinach and cilantro with water.

2. It must be smooth so blend it until it gets smoother.

3. Now add the left items and blend again. Enjoy.

Banana-Choc-Chai Smoothie

You guessed it. That is another variation on a style. If you want the Chai group of recipes you then will find that every one although virtually identical gives a completely different effect. And After all totally.

First blend

1 cup of water

1 couple of sunflower seeds

1 couple of almonds

Then add

1 frozen banana

2 tbsp chia gel

6 dried fruit chopped (figs and or apricots)

½ avocado

2 cups of mild greens in virtually any combination. Usage spinach, mizuna, chickweed, nice potato leaves or others from your own mild greens list ½ tsp of cinnamon, ¼ tsp of nutmeg, 1-2 tsp of vanilla, Dash of sea salt

Then as your final step add

¼ cup of raw cacao nibs

1 cup of ice

Banana Raspberry Yum

Remember that if you work with any frozen fruit then you'll probably need significantly more water and less ice. Fruit results in you focus on 1 cup of water to blend and add ice to get that pleasing coolness a smoothie appears to need! You can throw in a small number of almonds having a cup of milk if you don't possess almond milk. When in doubt or if there aren't nuts within the cupboard, use water. It'll be delicious.

1 cup almond milk (or additional nut milk, or add ¼ cup almonds and blend with water 1st))

1.5 cups raspberries (frozen)

2 bananas (fresh or frozen)

1 cup spinach

1 cup romaine (cos) lettuce (or 2 cups total mild greens of any combination)

¼ cup chopped mint leaves

Ice

Berrylicious

This is an excellent smoothie for the uninitiated and a simply great place to begin for children. They have a lot of berries and banana.

1 cup of water

1 cup raspberries (fresh or frozen)

1 cup various other berries (fresh or frozen)

2 bananas

2 cups spinach (or mild greens in virtually any combination)

Sea salt, cinnamon, and vanilla

Put ice and water for desired thickness and temperature

Pineapple Broccoli Sensation

Blended with the proper ingredients you can determine whether it's a taste to check or someone to become masked without anyone being the wiser. The broccoli with this smoothie enhances the different greens and helps decrease the acidity in the pineapple. It consistently scores a 9. Sweeter pineapples are always better in smoothies incidentally.

1 cup of water

1 medium tomato, chopped

2 cups mild greens (try romaine/cos or baby spinach)

½ cup broccoli florets

1 cup pineapple (no skin)

¼-1/3 cup cilantro (coriander) leaves and stems

Ice

Pineapple Dilly Dally

You should use lemon juice rather than lime if you want. It's optional to utilize ½ an avocado to 'smooth it up' a lot more.

1 cup of water

¼ cup dill

1 tbsp lime juice

1 tomato

1 cup kale

1 cup bok or Pak Choy (don't feel constrained. If you don't own kale and Choy, simply make use of 2 cups mild greens. Be sure you vary your green intake)

1.5 cups pineapple

OPTIONAL: ½ avocado

Increase ice and water for desired temperature and consistency

Herbal Ginger Beet

Even though I have an excellent blender, I do prefer to blend the carrot and beet initially with water to obtain a smoother consistency of the ultimate product. You should use any proportion of the two 2 cups of greens as mild and strong. Taste test thoroughly your leaves. Mustard can be quite strong particularly if you sip your smoothie as time passes. The spiciness appears to develop. The safer 'strong' greens, to begin with, are often watercress and rocket. Be brave, you're likely to find there are a great number of these recipes that taste surprisingly fantastic with strong greens.

First blend

We cup water

¼ cup beet chopped

¼ cup carrot chopped small

Bit ginger

Then add

1 cup mild greens (for eg: spinach, kale, Choy, sweet potato leaves)

1 cup strong greens (rocket, watercress or mustard leaves)

¼ cup cilantro/coriander

½ cup broccoli

1 cup of water

Finally

1 cup ice and blend again

Recommendations

To include taste bud drama, add cayenne and lime juice.

Vary the number of strong greens for your taste. Prefer mild greens?

Then use 2 cups.

Saladicious

This one's filled with many great ingredients, almost just like a liquid salad.

The sweetness is mild and originates from the beet and carrot. The essential smoothie is quite mild. Because it's greener and less nice it seems to get better for green smoothie aficionados. The parsley, ginger, and lime lift it. To get more taste bud action to add some cayenne and cumin.

First blend

1 cup of water

¼ cup beet chopped

¼ cup carrot chopped small

Bit ginger

Then add

½ avocado

1 cup mild greens (spinach, kale, Choy, sweet potato leaves)

1 cup strong greens (rocket, watercress or mustard leaves)

¼ cup cilantro/coriander

1 cup parsley

Sea salt

2 tbsp lime juice

1 cup ice and blend again

Recommendations

To green it up a lot more put in a stalk of celery or perhaps a cup of broccoli

Then add cayenne pepper and cumin

Salad Sunset

Nice and savory in a single. The pineapple does indeed an excellent job to

complement the vegetables here.

First blend

1 cup of water

¼ cup beet chopped

¼ cup carrot chopped small

Bit ginger

Then add

1 cup pineapple

½ avocado

2 cups greens (incorporating mild or more to at least one

1 cup strong greens)

¼ cup cilantro/coriander

¼ cup broccoli

Ice

Blue Bat

Blueberries always impart an excellent dark color to any smoothie. You may regard this one as a base to create additional recommended smoothie variations below.

1 cup of water

1 cup blueberries (frozen or fresh)

2 cups mild greens (get one of this choy, mizuna, cabbage)

1 kiwi fruit (with the hard end removed)

1 small tomato

Ice and blend

Recommendations

For spare sweetness then add apple, ½ cup pineapple or even a date or even to create different taste sensations: Add mint OR coriander/cilantro

Blueberry Pineapple Smoothie

The complement of greens within this smoothie comprises of celery, cilantro plus the mild green of your decision.

1 cup pineapple

2 tomatoes

1 cup blueberries (frozen or fresh)

¼ cup coriander

1 cup spinach leaves or other mild leafy green

1 stick celery chopped

1 squeeze of lemon to taste

Ice as required

Berry Packed Smoothie

The tang of raspberries, the color of blueberries along with the sweetness of bananas.

Blend first

1 cup of water

¼ cup (soaked) almonds

Then add

1 cup raspberries

¼ cup blueberries

1 banana

½ cup broccoli

1 small-medium tomato

1.5 cup spinach leaves

Ice

Just what A Lovely Pear

With this smoothie, I've recommended using kale. The others of the 2 cup greens component are mint. When I take advantage of any green I'll use a lot of the stalk as I could. Just eliminate woody ends. I don't believe it's sound policy to just utilize the leaves as you'll lose out on a whole lot of nourishment and fiber. It's all (in cases like this) good!

1 cup of water

1 pear

1 orange peeled

1 cup pineapple

½ cup mint

1.5 cup kale (or other mild green)

Ice as required

Tangy Tex Mex

The smoothness of avocado balanced with sweet, salty, and tangy flavors with some cilantro.

1 cup of water

½ cup pineapple

½ large avocado

2 tomatoes

½ cup red bell pepper

1.5 cups greens (your decision, mild or strong)

½ cup cucumber

¼ cup coriander

1 tbsp lime juice (add even more to improve the tang)

Pinch cayenne pepper (to taste)

Pinch sea salt

Ice

Dance towards the Beet

Orange provides a number of the liquid therefore I just added ½ cup normal water to start.

½ cup of water

1 orange

¼ cup beet

¼ - ½ cup parsley

2 cups greens according to taste. I take advantage of 1 cup mild (spinach, asparagus lettuce or chickweed) and 1 cup strong (watercress or rocket)

Ginger

1 cup ice

Mango Spice

Your kids give this thumbs up!

Blend first

1 cup of water

8 brazil nut products (or make use of a cup of nut milk or plain water)

Then add

½ avocado

2 cups mild greens (such as tatsoi or chickweed)

1 cup mango (frozen or fresh)

1 tsp cinnamon, ½ tsp nutmeg

Vanilla

1 cup ice

Recommendations

If you want more sweetness, add more mango or 2 bits of dried fruit. I love the feel beneath the tooth. You can sweeten with syrup or stevia although I tend towards fruit easily might help it.

Clove or cardamom powder can deepen the spice profile for you personally

Choc-Mango Spice

Has got the green light!

Blend first

1 cup of water

8 brazil nuts

(or make use of a cup of nut milk)

Then add

2 cups mild greens (in virtually any combination)

1 cup of frozen mango

½ avocado

Vanilla

1 tsp cinnamon, ½ tsp nutmeg

¼ cup raw cacao nibs (or some cacao powder to taste)

1 cup ice

Recommendations

If you want more sweetness, add ½ cup more mango or 2 bits of dried fruit.

Clove or cardamom powder are other handy spices that complement cinnamon and nutmeg.

Blue Eyes Smoothie

If you're fortunate to get fresh blueberries readily available you might throw in ½ cup of ice towards the blend. Correctly up there with good, taste
and score on top of that.

1 cup of water

1 cup blueberries (frozen or fresh)

1 apple

½ cup coriander

1 stalk celery

1.5 cups mild greens

Sea salt

Lemon juice to taste

Ice as you will need it!

Recommendation

To make a different experience add a small number of
mint

Vanilla Pudding Smoothie

This smoothie (which unbelievably more often than not
scores 10 out of 10) is filled with nutritious brazil nuts,
avocado, and undoubtedly a mountain of leafy greens. It'll
be thick so to make it drinkable, bring more drinking water
½ cup at the same time. I love to eat that one having a
spoon, just like a pudding dessert.

Initially blend the nuts and water. Then add the additional
ingredients.

½ cup brazil nuts

1 cup of water

2 dates (take away the pits obviously ;))

½ avocado

1.5 - 2 tsp vanilla

¼ tsp sea salt

2 cups mild greens (use spinach or chickweed)

Ice if you want it

Recommendation

Rather than dates add dried peaches or apricots for a lot more nutrition.

Soak them (adding soak water too) if you'd like them very smooth.

Carob Vanilla Spice Pudding Smoothie

OK, OK, so that it looks nearly the same as Vanilla Pudding, but that's simply on paper. However, it is different which is SO good you should know steps to make that one in its right.

Blend first

1 cup of water

½ cup cashews (soaked when you have them obtainable, dry can do)

3 dates (no stone. Or other dried fruit)

Then add

2 tbsp carob

1 small avocado, or ½ large

2 cups mild greens

¼ - ½ tsp cinnamon

Vanilla

Pinch sea salt

1 cup ice or as needed

Recommendation

Rather than dates add dried peaches or apricots for a lot more nutrition. Soak them (adding soak water too) if you'd like them very smooth.

Mint Vanilla Pudding Smoothie

If you wish to drink this delicious smoothie, keep adding water until you get the desired consistency. It's beautifully suitable utilizing a spoon and savoring every last mouthful.

First of all, blend the nuts and water. Then add the various other ingredients.

½ cup brazil nuts

1 cup of water

2 dates

½ avocado

1.5 - 2 tsp vanilla

¼ tsp salt

1 cup mild greens (use spinach or chickweed)

1 cup mint

Ice, if you will!

Recommendation

Rather than dates add dried peaches or apricots for a lot more nutrition.

Soak them (adding soak water too) if you'd like them very smooth.

Kiwi Vanilla Smoothie

What may I say? This cornucopia of interesting ingredients works out a delicious 10/10 scoring smoothie! If you don't have sprouts readily available just add a supplementary ½ cup of mild greens.

First blend:

A couple of almonds

1 cup of water

Then add

2 dates

1 tsp vanilla essence

2 kiwi

¼ tsp salt

1 cup kale (or mild greens)

½ cup broccoli

A couple of sprouts

Recommendation

Replace your dates with dried peaches or apricots for a lot more nourishment. Soak them (adding soak water too) if you'd like them very smooth.

Gleaming Green Spinach and Lettuce Smoothie

Yield: 2 glasses

Ingredients:

3 cups chopped romaine lettuce (or around 1 head)

2 cups chopped spinach leaves (about 50 % of a big bunch)

½ cup sliced celery

½ cup diced apples (about ½ mid-sized whole)

¼ cup diced pear (about 1 mid-sized whole)

½ cup sliced banana

½ tablespoon fresh lemon juice

1 cup of water

Preparation:

1. Wash all fruit and veggies completely before handling them.

2. Put romaine lettuce, spinach, and normal water together inside a blender.

Procedure at low speed until the mixture becomes smooth.

3. Bring celery, apple, and pear. Blend mixture at broadband.

4. Lastly, add the banana and lemon juice and puree until well blended.

5. Pour into glasses and serve fresh.

Variation:

Add ½ cup each of parsley and cilantro for a straight greener smoothie. Using stems are okay, but chop them so they don't ruin your blender or smoothie maker.

Supply an inch of ginger to recipe for a supplementary zing.

Smoothie fact:

This smoothie is 7 parts vegetables and 3 parts fruit, which means this can help you put more greens into your daily diet than you normally could in a single sitting.

This well-mixed green smoothie is simple to digest, which can make the body absorb more minerals and vitamins. Plus, this smoothie is usually amazingly filling, so that it could keep you from reaching for that carbohydrate packed snack merely to pacify your food cravings.

Vigour Booster Spinach and Collard Greens

Smoothie

Yield: 1 glass

Ingredients:

1 cup fresh spinach

1 cup fresh collard greens

4 whole mid-sized oranges

3 cups pineapple chunks

Preparation:

1. Squeeze out the juice from your oranges. Use this fresh juice as a liquid base for blending the spinach and collard greens.

Blend at slow speed until smooth.

2. Put the pineapples for the orange and greens mixture and blend at broadband until good mixed.

3. Pour and serve immediately.

Variation:

Need this smoothie to double like a cold thirst quencher? Add 6 ice cubes into the mix and blend until smooth.

Can't find collard greens? Take it easy by replacing using a cup of chopped kale.

Smoothie fact:

Packed with fruits & vegetables which are abundant with minerals, proteins, and vitamins A, C, E, and K, this smoothie is a surefire energy booster that may allow the body to operate at an optimal level. That's real, green, and mean energy within a glass!

Minty Papaya Green Smoothie

Yield: 1 glass

Ingredients:

3 cups spinach leaves

2 cups cubed ripe papaya

1 cup cubed pear

2 tablespoons goji berries (dried or fresh)

10 fresh leaves of mint

1 cup of filtered water

Preparation:

1. Pour water into a blender. Bring papaya first, accompanied by the pear, berries, and mint leaves. Add the spinach last.

2. Blend on broadband for approximately 30 seconds or before smoothie turns into a straight and creamy consistency.

3. Serve fresh.

Variation:

Substitute papaya with the same a part of a banana and you'll still possess a creamy smoothie.

Pour smoothie into an airtight container and chill within the refrigerator overnight to produce a refreshing morning smoothie meal replacement.

Smoothie fact:

This smoothie recipe packs within an abundance of protein, folate, magnesium, and potassium. Additionally, it is saturated in vitamins A, B1, B6, C, and K.

Apart from its high vitamins and minerals, ripe papaya can be an excellent creamy fruit base for your smoothie.

Green Piña Colada Smoothie

Yield: 4 glasses

Ingredients:

1 cup sliced dandelion greens

4 cups fresh ripe pineapple chunks

½ cup shredded coconut meat

4 tablespoons dried pitted dates

2 cups unsweetened coconut water

2 cups ice

Preparation:

1. Put all ingredients inside a blender. Be sure you place the liquid first as well as the greens last. Add ingredients among.

2. Blend on broadband until a creamy and smooth puree is achieved.

3. Pour into glasses and serve.

Variation:

For any nutty taste, add 4 tablespoons raw cashew nut products towards the recipe.

Be sure that you choose the best cashews (plump, uniform in color, smells nutty and sweet) and always soak them initially to eliminate enzyme inhibitors and make sure they are more digestible.

Smoothie fact:

Dandelion greens could be bitter when eaten raw, but adding this super green vegetable to the mix can make your smoothie taste enjoy it has alcohol in it.

On top of that, dandelion greens are reported to be the best detox and cleansing green since it is a superb liver cleanser.

Kiwi Green Smoothie

Yield: 1 glass

Ingredients:

1 cup cut kale leaves

1 cup sliced Romaine lettuce

1 cup cut Swiss chard leaves

½ cup sliced ripe bananas

½ kiwi fruit

Juice of ½ lemon

1 cup distilled water

1 teaspoon bee pollen

½ teaspoon maca powder

Preparation:

1. Wash all ingredients thoroughly. Prepare as directed inside the recipe.

2. Put all ingredients within a blender. Blend at broadband until smooth.

3. Pour right into a glass and serve immediately.

Variation:

Replace normal water with the same amount of unsweetened coconut water for extra alkaline within your green smoothie.

If kiwis aren't in season, substitute it with mango or papaya.

Smoothie fact:

Adding nutrition supplements like bee pollen and maca powder inside your green smoothie increase the health advantages that the body will get from your mix.

Minty Green Smoothie

Yield: 2 glasses

Ingredients:

1 cup sliced spinach leaves

10 pieces of mint leaves

2 whole pitted dates

2 tablespoons raw cashew butter

1 ½ cups distilled water

Preparation:

1. Put all ingredients inside a blender. Whiz on broadband until smooth.

2. Pour into glasses and serve immediately.

Variation:

Substitute pitted dates with 1 tablespoon of raw coconut nectar or raw agave nectar

Add 1 cup of ice for any cold treat

Smoothie fact:

Mint not merely triggers a sense of satiety (it certainly makes you look full!) but also helps flush out poisons from the digestive system. It also supports proper digestion by soothing the intestines and loosening intestinal muscles, thus relieving cramps along with other symptoms of the disturbed stomach.

Avocado Lime Smoothie

Yield: 1 glass

Ingredients:

1 cup young spinach leaves

½ cup sliced cucumber

½ avocado fruit

3 whole limes

Sweetener (honey, agave or stevia) to taste

6 pieces of ice

Preparation:

1. Wash fruits and vegetables thoroughly.

2. Pluck out the leaves from the spinach. Discard stems.

3. Without peeling, cut the cucumber into half-inch slices.

4. Remove the seed of the avocado. Utilizing a spoon, scoop out flesh through the peeling.

5. Peel and quarter limes.

6. Inside a blender, place cucumber, avocado, spinach, and lime. Supply ice and preferred amount of sweetener.

7. Blend all ingredients until smooth.

8. Pour right into a glass and drink fresh.

Variation:

Put ½ teaspoon cinnamon powder to include zing in your smoothie.

If you discover your smoothie too thick, add ½ cup of cold distilled water and blend again before serving.

Smoothie fact:

The high pH degree of limes helps balance the body's alkaline amounts and protects it from diseases and infections.

Tropical Kale Green Smoothie

Yield: 1 glass

Ingredients:

1 cup kale leaves

1 mid-sized apple

1 mid-sized avocado

¼ lemon fruit

1 tablespoon sliced ginger

A pinch of salt

½ cup distilled water

Preparation:

1. Rinse kale in running water. Tear leaves apart.

2. Without peeling, core, and segment apples.

3. Cut avocado into halves, remove seed and scoop out flesh utilizing a tablespoon.

4. Peel the lemon and remove seeds.

5. Peel ginger and cut into thin slices.

6. Put all ingredients within a blender. Whiz on broadband until well mixed and smooth.

7. Pour right into a tall glass and revel in!

Variation:

Use limes rather than lemon to get a slightly different taste.

Rather than adding a sweetener like honey or agave nectar, you may make this smoothie taste sweeter with the addition of more apples.

Rather than avocado, you can even use an equal part banana with this recipe.

Almond Swirl

1 cup almond milk

2 ripe peaches, pits removed, cut into chunks

½ cup kale, chopped

1-2 drops stevia

1 tsp. pure vanilla extract

½ tsp. pure almond extract

6 ice cubes

Combine all ingredients inside a blender and procedure good until smooth and creamy. Serve chilled. Serves 2.

Amazon Kicker

1 cup fresh apple juice

½ cup frozen unsweetened the acai berry

½ cup spinach

1 cup fresh or frozen strawberries

1 medium frozen banana, cut into chunks

4 ice cubes

Combine all ingredients within a blender and operation good until smooth and creamy. Serve chilled. Serves 2.

Apple Spice

2 cups natural yogurt

1 cup cut apple

1 cup baby spinach, packed

½ tsp. ground cinnamon or apple pie spice

½ cup fresh orange juice

Combine all ingredients inside a blender and method good until smooth and creamy. Serve chilled. Serves 2.

Avocado Cream

½ cup almond milk

1 avocado, peeled and seeded

1 couple of spinach

2 Tbsp. fresh lemon juice

2-3 drops stevia

1 tsp. pure vanilla extract

1 tsp. organic lemon peel, freshly grated

6 ice cubes

Combine all ingredients within a blender and course of action good until smooth and creamy. Serve chilled. Serves 1.

Aztec Chili Cacao

1½ cups almond milk

½ cup spinach or chopped kale

1 banana, peeled and cut into chunks

½ vanilla bean

¼ jalapeño pepper, seeds removed if you don't like hot foods

½ tsp. cinnamon

1-2 Tbsp. cacao

Stevia drops to taste

6-8 ice cubes

Combine all ingredients inside a blender and approach well until smooth and creamy. Serve chilled. Serves 1-2.

Berries 'n' Cream

1 cup strawberries with caps

1 banana, peeled, and cut into chunks

1 cup natural yogurt

½ cup loosely packed flat-leaf parsley

3-4 drops stevia (optional)

6 ice cubes

Combine all ingredients within a blender and procedure good until smooth and creamy. Serve chilled. Serves 2.

Celery Green Smoothie

1 stalk celery, sliced thin

4 True Ripe Bananas

A small number of Baby Spinach

1 cup Ice Water or ICE

Add each one of these ingredients for the blender and puree until smooth.

Collard Green smoothie

4 oz. Coconut Water

1 Frozen Banana

1 cup Blueberries

1 cup Seedless Grapes

A small number of Collard Greens, with no stems and stalk.

½ cup Ice Water or ice

Add each one of these ingredients towards the blender and puree until it is a smoothie.

This one is good. Everything combination of flavors would produce a very tasty lunch.

Mango Green Smoothie

1 Frozen Banana

1 Mango, sliced

2 good handfuls of Baby Spinach

1cup Ice Water

Add each one of these ingredients for the blender and puree until smooth

Spicy Delicious Green Smoothie

½ cup of Pure Vanilla Almond Milk

1 Banana

Dash of Cinnamon

1 couple of Spinach

1 tablespoon Whey Powder

1 cup Ice

Add each one of these ingredients towards the blender and puree until smooth.

All-Purpose Green Smoothie

1 Banana

1 sliced Apple

1 sliced pear

1 stalk Celery, break up

½ Lemon

2 handfuls of Spinach

1 handful Romaine Lettuce

Little Parsley

Little Cilantro

1 cup Ice

Add all of the ingredients for the blender then squeeze the lemon over it. Puree until it is smooth.

Green tea extract Smoothie

1 cup GREEN TEA EXTRACT

1 Carrot

1 Banana

2 handfuls kale (using the no stems or stalk)

Few ICE

Add all of the ingredients towards the blender and puree until smooth. That one is a superb decision for lunch.

Lemon Cucumber Green Smoothie

1 Cucumber

1 Pear, sliced

4 Celery Stalks

1 peeled Lemon

½ cup Ice Water

Add each one of these ingredients for the blender and puree until they may be smooth.

A perfect selection for lunch; that one will provide you with the energy you will need for all of those other afternoons.

Cashew Green Smoothie

1 cup Coconut Water

½ cup Cashews

1 Banana

2 Dates

1 tablespoon Flax Seed

One couple of Spinach

Add all of the ingredients towards the blender and puree until it is smooth. That one is usually delicious plus the cashews give it something special. A great choice for lunch

Orange Green Smoothie

1 Banana

5 Large Strawberries

½ cup Peeled Orange

½ cup sliced Apple

Little Flax Seed

2 handfuls of Spinach

1 cup Ice Water

Mix all of the ingredients into the blender and puree until smooth. That one is wonderful and ideal for lunch.

Fruit and Green Smoothie

1 small container Plain Greek Yogurt

1/2cup Natural Protein Powder

½ cup Blueberries

½ cup Peaches, sliced

½ cup Pineapple, sliced

½ cup Strawberries

½ cup Mango, sliced

1 couple of Kale (remove stem and stalks)

½ cup Ice Water

Add each one of these ingredients for the blender and puree until smooth. That one is out of the world.

Ginger Green Smoothie

Small couple of parsley

1 Cucumber, sliced

1 peeled Lemon

1 inch of Ginger Root

1 cup Frozen Apples

1 handful Kale (minus the stems and stalks)

½ cup Ice Water

Mix each one of these ingredients into the blender and puree until smooth. That one is great. Each one of these ingredients is wonderful together. Good choice for lunch

Melon Green Shake

½ cup Black Cherries pitted

1 Banana

Little couple of Kale, break up

½ cup Blueberries

½ cup Green Melon

½ cup Coconut Water

½ cup ICE

Add each one of these ingredients towards the blender and puree until it is smooth. That one is great. All of the flavors are wonderful together.

Almond Coconut Yogurt Green Smoothie

1 cup Almond Coconut Yogurt

A couple of Cilantro

A couple of Spinach

Avocado, sliced

1 cup Blueberries, Strawberries or Raspberries

1 Mango, sliced

½ cup Coconut Water

Pinch of Sea Salt

Ice Water (just as much as you need to obtain the thickness for your taste)

Add all of the ingredients for the blender and puree until smooth. Add water as needed. That is a delicious green smoothie with an excellent taste. All of this combination of flavors is a delicacy to drink. This recipe makes enough for 4 large smoothies.

Refreshing Green Smoothie

1 cup Pineapple, break up

1 Frozen Banana, break up

1 Mango, sliced

½ cup Ice Water

Handful Baby Spinach

Add all of the ingredients towards the blender and puree until smooth. That one is delicious and refreshing. That is a fantastic choice for lunch.

These recipes are very easy and the greatest thing is you could alter any ingredients to fit your taste. So long as you supply organic fruit plus some sort of vegetable greens that can be healthy you should use anything. Put ice or ice water as necessary for the thickness you like. It generally does not consider any time whatsoever no matter how busy a person they have time to get ready these recipes.

Banana Swiss Chard Smoothie with Lime

2 Fresh or Frozen Bananas

3 cups Swiss Chard

½ of the Lime

1 cup Ice

Directions

Remove is due to Swiss chard and discard.

Roughly chop Swiss chard.

Peel and segment half a lime into small pieces. This can help when blending ingredients.

Slice bananas into ½ inch slices.

Within a blender add bananas, Swiss chard, lime, and ice.

Blend on the highest speed until smooth.

Spinach and Flaxseed Protein Smoothie

1 A couple of Spinach

1tsp. of Flax Seeds (ground)

1¼ cup Coconut Water

½ cup Plain Greek Yogurt

½ scoop Vanilla Protein Powder

1 cup Ice

Directions

Roughly chop spinach.

Bring all ingredients to the blender.

Blend until smooth and well mixed.

Mint Chocolate Smoothie with Spinach

1 cup Milk (Skim, 2 % or Entire is okay)

2 handfuls of Baby Spinach

1 scoop Chocolate Protein Powder

1 scoop Cocoa Powder

Mint Leaves (crushed)

2-3 drops Peppermint Extract

5 Ice Cubes

Directions

Crush mint leaves.

Contribute all ingredients into a blender. Blend until smooth and creamy.

Strawberry Banana Protein Smoothie with Spinach

½ of any Banana

1 cup Skim Milk

1 cup Fresh or Frozen Strawberries

1 scoop of Vanilla Protein Powder

1 couple of Baby Spinach

3 Ice Cubes

Directions

Supply all ingredients into a blender.

Blend until smooth.

Apple Cinnamon Smoothie with Romaine Lettuce

1 couple of Romaine Lettuce

1 Banana

1 cup Water

1 cup Ice

½ teaspoon Ground Cinnamon or even to taste

2 Apples

Directions

Chop lettuce, banana, and apples.

Put all ingredients to a blender.

Blend on high till smooth.

Green Peanut Butter and Banana Smoothie

1 cup Almond Milk

1 tablespoon Peanut Butter

1 Frozen Banana

1 handful of Baby Spinach

Directions

Thinly slice the frozen banana.

Bring all ingredients and blend on high until smooth.

Protein Pear and Kale Smoothie

1½ cups Water

2 cups Kale

2 ripe Pears

1 Frozen Banana

1 scoop Protein Powder

¼ Avocado

1 tbsp Flax Seed

1 cup Ice

¼ cup Cilantro

Directions

Roughly chop kale.

Slice frozen banana

Core pears and chop into small pieces.

Blend kale, water, and herbs for on high for approximately one minute.

Put remaining ingredients and blend on high for approximately one minute or until smooth.

Mint and Pear Smoothie with Ginger

2 handfuls of Kale or Spinach

1 ½ cup of Water

1 Pear

1 little bit of Ginger (Fresh)

Mint (to taste)

1 tsp. Flaxseed

Directions

Remove is due to kale.

Remove the core and cut the pear into pieces.

Increase kale and drinking water into a blender.

Blend on high until greens are dissolved into water.

Add more flaxseed and blend until divided into the mixture.

Insert pear ginger and mint.

Blend until smooth.

Green Grape and Pumpkin Smoothie

2 cups Green Grapes (Seedless)

1 Pear

1 cup Spinach

½ cup Frozen Pumpkin Purée

¾ cup Coconut Water

Ice Cubes

2 tbsp. Avocado

1 Pear, cored and chopped

Add all ingredients to the blender. Blend on high until smooth.

Fruity Green Smoothie

6 Large Strawberries

½ Banana

1 Large Orange

1/3 cup Simple Greek Yogurt

2 cups Spinach

1 cup Ice

Directions

Cut strawberries into chunks. Remove green leaves.

Slice 1 / 2 of banana into ½ inch pieces.

Peel and segment orange

Put all ingredients into a blender.

Blend until smooth.

Mean Greeny Juice

Ingredients:

Celery- 3 stalks

Cucumbers- 2 piece

Spinach- 5 fresh leaves

Parsley- ½ cup

Wheatgrass- 3 inch

Drinking water- 2 cup

Directions:

1. Pour everything simultaneously in blender

2. Blend for at least three minutes.

3. Enjoy

Veggie Smoothie

Ingredients:

Celery- 3 stalks

Carrots- 2 piece

Red Beet- ½ piece

Spinach- 5 leaves

Alfalfa sprouts- ½ cup

Wheatgrass- 3 inch

Normal water- 2 cups

Directions:

1. Pour everything simultaneously in blender

2. Blend for at least three minutes.

3. Enjoy

Grass of Apple

Ingredients:

Apples- 3 piece

Wheatgrass- 3 inch

Drinking water- 2 cups

Directions:

1. Pour everything simultaneously in blender

2. Blend for at least three minutes.

3. Enjoy

Grass of Wheat

Ingredients:

Oranges- 2 pieces

Banana- 1 piece

Berry- ½ cup

Wheat Grass- 2 inch

Ice Cubes- 1 cup

Directions:

1. Pour everything simultaneously in blender

2. Blend for at least three minutes.

3. Enjoy

Grass of Orange

Ingredients:

Orange- 2 piece

Carrots- 2 piece

Wheat Grass- 3inch

Directions:

1. Pour everything simultaneously in blender

2. Blend for at least three minutes.

3. Enjoy

Wintergreen smoothie

Ingredients:

Apples- 4 piece

Pears- 2 piece

Celery- 2 sticks

Kale- large bunch

Watercress- 1 small bunch

Chili- 1 small size

Directions:

1. Pour everything simultaneously in blender

2. Blend for at least three minutes.

3. Enjoy

Spring with Green Smoothie

Ingredients:

Lettuce- 2 heads

Spring greens- 4 cups

Cucumber- 1 piece

A sprig of parsley- 1 small piece

Lemon juice- 1 piece

Directions:

1. Pour everything simultaneously in blender

2. Blend for at least three minutes.

3. Enjoy

Summer with Green Smoothie

Ingredients:

cucumber- ½ piece

Honeydew melon- ½ piece

Seedless grapes- small bunch

kiwi- 2 pieces

Spinach- 2 cup

Mint- 1 small cup

Lemon juice- ½ cup

Directions:

1. Pour everything simultaneously in blender

2. Blend for at least three minutes.

3. Enjoy

Fall in love Smoothie

Ingredients:

Apples- 3 pieces

Cucumber- 1 piece

Celery- 3 sticks

Grapes- small bunch

Honeydew- 1 large pice

Basil- a small sprig

Directions:

1. Pour everything simultaneously in blender

2. Blend for at least three minutes.

3. Enjoy

Carrot with Spinach

Ingredients:

Carrots- 5 piece

Spinach- 1 cup

Directions:

1. Pour everything simultaneously in blender

2. Blend for at least three minutes.

3. Enjoy

Raw Spinach Fun Smoothie

Ingredients:

Spinach- 1 bunch

Raw honey- 1 teaspoon

Directions:

1. Pour everything simultaneously in blender

2. Blend for at least three minutes.

3. Enjoy

Spinach with Tomato

Ingredients:

Spinach- 1 cup

Tomato- 4 pieces

Directions:

1. Pour everything simultaneously in blender

2. Blend for at least three minutes.

3. Enjoy

Spinach with Beet Carrot

Ingredients:

Beet- ½ with top

Carrot- 3 piece

Spinach- ½ cup

Directions:

1. Pour everything simultaneously in blender

2. Blend for at least three minutes.

3. Enjoy

Cucumber and Spinach mix

Ingredients:

carrots- 4 pieces

apple- 1 piece

Cucumber- ¼ piece

Spinach- 1 cup

Directions:

1. Pour everything simultaneously in blender

2. Blend for at least three minutes.

3. Enjoy

Carnival on Ice

½ cup fresh apple juice (1 apple, juiced)

1 cup fresh or frozen blueberries, rinsed if fresh

1 frozen banana, cut into chunks

1 green leaf lettuce, chopped

½ cup raw cashews

½ tsp. pure vanilla extract

6 ice cubes

Combine all ingredients inside a blender and procedure good until smooth and creamy. Serve chilled. Serves 2.

Carob Classic

1 cup almond or coconut milk

½ cup spinach

2 Tbsp. carob powder (cocoa powder could be substituted)

1 tsp. pure vanilla extract

1 frozen or fresh banana, cut into chunks

Pour the milk right into a blender, and add the spinach, carob, vanilla, and banana. Process until smooth and creamy. Pour right into a glass and serve at the earliest opportunity. Serves 1.

Chai Green

1 cup almond milk

1 banana, cut into chunks

1 cup sliced greens of preference

½ tsp. ground cinnamon

1/8 tsp. ground cardamom

1/8 tsp. ground coriander

1/8 tsp. ground cloves

1/8 tsp. ground black pepper

5-6 drops stevia or 1 Tbsp. honey

6 ice (or 6 ice of frozen chai green tea extract)

Combine all ingredients within a blender and operation good until smooth and creamy. Serve chilled. Serves 2.

Cherie's Green Morning Blend

½ English cucumber, peeled if not organic and cut into chunks

1 avocado, peeled, seeded, and cut into quarters

1 cup loosely packed baby spinach

Juice of just one 1 lime

1 Tbsp. green powder of preference (optional)

2-3 Tbsp. ground almonds (optional)

Combine all ingredients inside a blender and blend well. Sprinkle ground almonds at the top, as preferred. Serves 1.

Chia Mia

10 raw almonds

1 Tbsp. raw sunflower seeds

1 Tbsp. chia seeds

1 Tbsp. sesame seeds

1 Tbsp. flaxseeds

1 cup pineapple juice (juice one-quarter pineapple, if producing fresh)

1 cup cut parsley

½ cup almond milk

½ tsp. pure vanilla extract

1 Tbsp. protein powder (optional)

6 ice cubes

Place the nuts, seeds, and pineapple juice within a bowl. Cover and soak overnight. Place the nut and seed mixture using the juice inside a blender and bring the parsley, milk, vanilla, protein powder (if using), and ice.

Blend on broadband until smooth. This drink is a piece chewy due to the nut products and seeds. Serves 2.

Note: To kill molds, add ½ tsp. ascorbic acid to juice, then add nuts and soak overnight.

Chocolate Chimps

1 banana, peeled and cut into chunks

1 Tbsp. cocoa or powdered cacao

1 Tbsp. peanut butter or almond butter

½ cup loosely packed baby spinach

½ cup almond milk

1-2 drops stevia

6 ice cubes

Place all ingredients within a blender and method until smooth and creamy.

Pour into glasses and serve chilled. Serves 2.

Cocoa Cabana

1 cup almond milk

1½ cups frozen banana, cut into chunks

1 cup chard, chopped

3 Tbsp. unsweetened cocoa powder

½ tsp. cinnamon

Pour the milk right into a blender and add the frozen banana chunks, chard, cocoa powder, and cinnamon. Blend until smooth. Serves 2.

Coconut Creamsicle

1 cup of coconut milk

1 orange, peeled, cut into chunks

½ cup grated coconut, lightly packed

½ cup loosely packed baby spinach

2 tsp. pure vanilla extract

4-5 drops stevia

6 ice cubes

Place all ingredients inside a blender and course of action until smooth and creamy.

Pour into glasses and serve chilled. Serves 2.

Simple fun with Green Smoothie

Ingredients:

Normal water- 1 cup

Banana- 1 piece

Spinach- 1 cup

The Directions are going to be the same for following Smoothies. Here that's:

1. You must take all of the ingredients and you must wash them properly.

2. Then simply add everything to your blender simultaneously

3. Blend for 3-4 minutes.

4. Consider it out and use ice cubes to create it cold.

5. Enjoy

Smoothie of Aloe Vera

Ingredients:

Coconut oil- 1 cup

Aloe Vera leaf- ½ cup

Blueberry- ½ cup

Frozen Mango- ½ cup

Coconut oil- ½ tsp

Basil- 1 handful

Stevia- optional

The Directions are going to be the same for following Smoothies. Here that's:

1. You must take all of the ingredients and you must wash them properly.

2. Then simply add everything to your blender simultaneously

3. Blend for 3-4 minutes.

4. Have it out and make use of ice cubes to create it cold.

5. Enjoy

Smoothie of Skin

Ingredients:

Drinking water- 1 cup

Aloe Vera leaf- 1 piece

Avocado- ¼ piece

Kiwi- 1 piece

Blueberry- ½ cup

Coconut oil- 1 tsp

Salt- 1 pinch

Honey- 1 tsp

The Directions are going to be the same for following Smoothies. Here that's:

1. You must take all of the ingredients and you must wash them properly.

2. Then simply add everything to your blender simultaneously

3. Blend for 3-4 minutes.

4. Require it out and employ ice cubes to create it cold.

5. Enjoy

Smoothie of Aloe

Ingredients:

Normal water- 1 cup

Aloe vera leaf- 1 medium piece

Spinach- 1 cup

Blueberry- ½ cup

Coconut oil- 1 tsp

Celtic Sea Salt- 1 dash

Stevia- optional

The Directions are going to be the same for following Smoothies. Here that's:

1. You must take all of the ingredients and you must wash them properly.

2. Then simply add everything to your blender simultaneously

3. Blend for 3-4 minutes.

4. Bring it out and work with ice cubes to create it cold.

5. Enjoy

Strawberry Fun

Ingredients:

Almond Milk- 1 cup

Diced aloe gel- ½ cup

Strawberry- ½ cup

Banana- ½ piece

Ice cube- 5 piece

Honey- optional

The Directions are going to be the same for following Smoothies. Here that's:

1. You must take all of the ingredients and you must wash them properly.

2. Then simply add everything to your blender simultaneously

3. Blend for 3-4 minutes.

4. Choose it and use ice cubes to create it cold.

5. Enjoy

Lemonade with Aloe Vera

Ingredients:

Drinking water- 1 cup

Avocado- ½ piece

Aloe vera- 1 medium piece

Lemon- ½ piece

Lime- ½ piece

Coconut oil- 1 tsp

Celtic salt- 1 dash

Honey- 1tsp

The Directions are going to be the same for following Smoothies. Here that's:

1. You must take all of the ingredients and you must wash them properly.

2. Then simply add everything to your blender simultaneously

3. Blend for 3-4 minutes.

4. Consider it and make use of ice cubes to make it cold.

5. Enjoy

Superfood Smoothie

Ingredients:

Normal water- 1 cup

Banana- 1 piece

Blueberry- ½ cup

Spinach- 1 cup

Kale- ½ cup

Coconut oil- 1 tsp

Spirulina- 1 tsp

Cinnamon- ¼ tsp

Maple syrup- optional

The Directions are going to be the same for following Smoothies. Here that's:

1. You must take all of the ingredients and you must wash them properly.

2. Then simply add everything to your blender simultaneously

3. Blend for 3-4 minutes.

4. Have it out and employ ice cubes to create it cold.

5. Enjoy

Mean Green Smoothie

Ingredients:

Drinking water- 1 cup

Lemon juice- ½ cup

Banana- 1 piece

Kale- 1 cup

Spirulina- 1 tsp

Chlorella- 1 tsp

Celtic sea salt- 1dash

Ice cubes- 3-5 piece

The Directions are going to be the same for following Smoothies. Here that's:

1. You must take all of the ingredients and you must wash them properly.
2. Then simply add everything to your blender simultaneously
3. Blend for 3-4 minutes.
4. Require it out and work with ice cubes to create it cold.
5. Enjoy

Basil Smoothie with Strawberry

Ingredients:

Drinking water- 1 cup

Frozen Banana- 1 piece

Strawberry- ½ cup

Basil Leaves- 10 piece

Ice cubes- 6 piece

Stevia- optional

The Directions are going to be the same for following Smoothies. Here that's:

1. You must take all of the ingredients and you must wash them properly.

2. Then simply add everything to your blender simultaneously

3. Blend for 3-4 minutes.

4. Consider it and use ice cubes to create it cold.

5. Enjoy

Basil Berry Smoothie

Ingredients:

Normal water- 1 cup

Banana- 1 piece

Spinach- 1 cup

Basil Leaves- 8 pieces

Frozen berries- 1 cup

Coconut oil- 1 tsp

Cinnamon- ¼ tsp

Stevia- optional

The Directions are going to be the same for following Smoothies. Here that's:

1. You must take all of the ingredients and you must wash them properly.

2. Then simply add everything to your blender simultaneously

3. Blend for 3-4 minutes.

4. Have it out and make use of ice cubes to create it cold.

5. Enjoy

Awesome fun with Aloe Vera

Ingredients:

Coconut milk- 1 cup

Aloe Vera- 1 cup

Blueberry- ½ cup

Mango chunks- ½ cup

Coconut oil- ½ tsp

Basil- 1 handful

Stevia- optional

The Directions are going to be the same for following Smoothies. Here that's:

1. You must take all of the ingredients and you must wash them properly.

2. Then simply add everything to your blender simultaneously

3. Blend for 3-4 minutes.

4. Require it out and employ ice cubes to make it cold.

5. Enjoy

Cilantro of Tropical Smoothie

Ingredients:

Drinking water- 1 cup

Cilantro- ½ cup

Pineapple- 1 cup

Mango- 1 cup

Lime juice- ½ cup

Celtic sea salt- 1 dash

The Directions are going to be the same for following Smoothies. Here that's:

1. You must take all of the ingredients and you must wash them properly.

2. Then simply add everything to your blender simultaneously

3. Blend for 3-4 minutes.

4. Bring it out and work with ice cubes to make it cold.

5. Enjoy

Smoothie of Cilantro Recipe

Ingredients:

Normal water- 1 cup

Banana- 1 piece

Cilantro- ½ cup

Lime juice- ½ cup

Celtic sea salt- 1 dash

Honey- 1 dash

The Directions are going to be the same for following Smoothies. Here that's:

1. You must take all of the ingredients and you must wash them properly.

2. Then simply add everything to your blender simultaneously

3. Blend for 3-4 minutes.

4. Choose it and use ice cubes to make it cold.

5. Enjoy

Fruity Green Smoothie

Yield: 1 glass

Ingredients:

½ cup chopped kale leaves

½ cup baby spinach leaves

½ cup berries (raspberry or strawberry)

1 cup sliced ripe banana

1 cup pear cubes

1 cup distilled water

Preparation:

1. Pour drinking water, kale, and spinach inside a blender. Whiz until smooth.

2. Bring remaining ingredients and continue blending until smooth.

3. Pour right into a glass and serve immediately.

Variation:

Top with a dash of cinnamon for an extra kick.

If you'd like your smoothie cold, only use ½ cup of water and add ½ cup of ice into the blend.

Smoothie fact:

It is nice to utilize berries within your green smoothie because they're saturated in antioxidants, which slows growing older by blocking free radicals from your body's system.

Green Coconut Smoothie

Yield: 1 glass

Ingredients:

1 cup sliced kale leaves

1 cup sliced ripe bananas

1 teaspoon raw honey

1 cup of coconut meat

1 cup of coconut water

½ cup ice

Preparation:

1. Inside a blender, mix all ingredients until smooth.

2. Pour right into a glass and serve immediately.

Variation:

To make this smoothie a lot more nutritious, put 2 tablespoons of organic green barley powder and 1 tablespoon of chia seeds.

Smoothie fact:

Coconut is simple to digest because fewer enzymes are needed to break it down, thus improving the stomach's capability to absorb nutrients and vitamins.

Banana Avocado Green Smoothie

Yield: 1 glass

Ingredients:

1 cup baby spinach

1 cup Swiss chard leaves

1 cup unripe banana chunks

½ mid-sized cucumber

½ avocado

1 whole lime

½ cup young coconut meat

1 cup unsweetened coconut water

Preparation:

1. Wash spinach, Swiss chard, and cucumber thoroughly in running water. Chop the leaves and slice the cucumber into 1-inch cubes.

2. Peel bananas and cut into 1-inch slices.

3. Scoop out the flesh from the avocado. Discard the seed.

4. Peel the lime and quarter.

5. Within a blender, mix spinach, Swiss chard, and coconut water until smooth.

6. Contribute remaining ingredients and blend until smooth and mixed thoroughly.

7. Pour right into a tall glass and revel in.

Variation:

Supply 3-5 mint leaves into the blend for an extra punch and cooling effect.

If you'd like your smoothie cold, chill within the refrigerator before drinking.

To sweeten the smoothie, put in a little bit of honey or mix a mid-sized cored and cubed red apple when blending.

Smoothie fact:

Raw bananas have significantly more resistant starch than ripe ones. Resistant starch can be a crucial element in weight loss since it inhibits digestion in the tiny intestines and helps block the conversion of carbohydrates.

Green Milk Smoothies

Tropical Green Kale Smoothie

Yield: 1 glass

Ingredients:

3 cups chopped kale leaves

1 whole mid-sized mango

½ cup sliced banana

½ lime fruit

1 cup unsweetened coconut milk

Preparation:

1. Wash and prepare all ingredients. Peel the mango, take away the seed and slice into 2-inch cubes. Juice the lime fruit.

2. Pour coconut milk into the blender. Add mango, banana, and lime juice. Add kale leaves last.

3. Blend all ingredients on broadband until smoothie reaches a creamy consistency (This will need about 30 seconds to process).

4. Pour right into a glass and serve fresh.

Variation:

Serve chilled or higher crushed ice for any refreshing drink perfect during hot days.

Do with no ice but make use of chilled or frozen chunks of mangoes instead. For any surprisingly cool twist, usually do not puree the mangoes and put the mango chunks right before serving.

Smoothie fact:

The tropical flavors of coconut, mango, and lime can make you imagine a location beneath the sun and increase your mood. This smoothie recipe also provides a powerful dose of vitamins, minerals, and dietary fibers.

Spinach Yogurt Smoothie

Yield: 2 glasses

Ingredients:

2 cups chopped spinach leaves

1 large whole orange

½ cup sliced bananas

1/3 cup strawberries

1/3 cup natural yogurt

1 cup ice

Preparation:

1. Peel oranges and divide into segments. Remove seeds if you will find any.

2. Put all ingredients within a blender. Puree until smooth.

3. Pour into glasses and serve immediately.

Variation:

Although this recipe demands strawberries, you should use other kinds of berries, too. Be not afraid, experiment!

Smoothie fact:

This smoothie is a superb post-workout or morning drink energy booster, because of the orange and berries in it. You can also drink only a glass of the smoothie and store the rest of the portion within an airtight container inside your refrigerator or freezer to get a later drink. Remember to thaw your smoothie through the freezer thirty minutes before you want to drink it.

Green Lime Pie Smoothie

Yield: 1 glass

Ingredients:

2 tablespoons lime juice

1 teaspoon lime zest

1 cup sliced ripe bananas

¼ teaspoon pure vanilla extract (alcohol-free)

1 tablespoon sunflower butter

2 cups shredded spinach leaves

1 entire pitted date

1 cup unsweetened nondairy milk

4 ice cubes

Preparation:

1. Prepare all ingredients.

2. Put everything inside a blender and whiz until smooth.

3. Pour right into a tall glass and serve immediately.

Variation:

To make this dessert smoothie more a lot more enticing, top with whipped cream and graham cracker bits.

Use strawberries or blueberries rather than lime for the different taste.

Smoothie fact:

Green smoothies may also serve as a dessert with the proper mixture of sweetness from 100 % natural ingredients like fruits. Usually do not mind the spinach because even though it offers a goblin green color for your smoothie, its slight taste is going to be masked from the fruits you blend it with.

Tropical Green Blast Smoothie

Yield: 1 glass

Ingredients:

2 cups spinach leaves

1 cup diced banana

1/3 cup diced ripe mangoes

1/3 cup pineapple chunks

¼ cup of orange juice

Preparation:

1. In this specific order, put spinach, banana, mango, pineapple, and orange juice inside the blender. Blend until ingredients are mixed (this will need about 90 minutes on broadband).

2. Put milk and blend again until mixed fully and smoothly.

3. Pour right into a glass and revel in.

Variation:

Put in a sprig of parsley (approximately 3 complete leaves) to include zing in your smoothie.

Smoothie fact:

When working with milk within your smoothie recipe, it's best not to employ dairy milk- even when it's low-fat- when using acidic fruits like pineapple and orange since it may bring about curdling. It is advisable to work with soy or coconut milk when working with acidic fruits.

Caramel Banana Green Smoothie

Yield: 1 glass

Ingredients:

1 cup spinach

1 cup sliced bananas

1 tablespoon caramel (store-bought)

1 tablespoon walnuts

½ cup of coconut milk

½ cup nondairy milk (soya, oat, almond, hemp or rice)

Preparation:

1. Put spinach, coconut milk, and non-dairy milk right into a blender.

Blend until thoroughly mixed.

2. Bring bananas, caramel, and walnuts. Blend until smooth.

3. Pour right into a tall glass and serve.

Variation:

To make this smoothie right into a cold drink, add ½ cup ice before blending or refrigerate before serving.

Produce your healthy caramel by boiling apple juice and putting it right into a simmer until it caramelizes.

Smoothie fact:

Spinach is a versatile green that's healthy yet mild in taste. When you have your own favorite fruit smoothie recipe, just add 1 cup of spinach for every glass of yield to carefully turn it right into a green smoothie.

Mango Spinach Green Smoothie

Yield: 1 glass

Ingredients:

1 cup spinach leaves

1/2 cup fresh ripe mango chunks

½ tablespoon linseeds

2 tablespoons desiccated coconut

2 tablespoons raisins

½ cup oat milk (could be substituted with any non-dairy milk)

½ cup of water

Preparation:

1. Blend spinach, oat milk, and water together until mixed well.

2. Add mangoes, linseeds, desiccated coconut, and raisins and blend on broadband until the mixture becomes smooth.

3. Pour right into a tall glass and serve.

Variation:

Supply ½ cup instant oats towards the recipe to produce a more filling smoothie.

Put ½ cup ice for just a cooler alternative.

Smoothie fact:

Mangoes are an unsung hero in weight loss. Filled with a lot more than 20 minerals and vitamins that protect your body against diseases, mangoes certainly are a rich way to obtain fiber and present a sense of fullness within the belly. Plus, it tastes deliciously nice so it can help you slim down without depriving yourself of the nice stuff.

Zucchini Vanilla Green Smoothie

Yield: 1 glass

Ingredients:

1 cup cut zucchini

1 cup baby spinach

1 small banana

2 tablespoons pecan nuts

2 tablespoons pitted dates

1 cup nondairy milk

½ teaspoon pure vanilla extract

A pinch of salt

Preparation:

1. Wash zucchini and spinach thoroughly. Without peeling, slice zucchini into half-inch thickness.

2. Peel the banana and cut into half-inch slices.

3. Put zucchini, spinach, vanilla extract, and milk within a blender and procedure until smooth. Bring all of the remaining ingredients and blend on broadband until smooth.

4. Pour right into a tall glass and drink.

Variation:

For a far more filling smoothie, add 1 cup of quinoa or oats into the recipe.

Need a cooler smoothie? Add ½ cup ice or ½ cup cool water into the blend.

Smoothie fact:

Zucchini supports weight loss since it is packed filled with important nutrients, dietary fibers, antioxidants, and vitamins A and C. Even though, it is lower in calories, this means it truly is a good replacement for filling you up.

No-Fruit Green Smoothie

Yield: 1 glass

Ingredients:

1 cup spinach

½ cup oats

½ teaspoon vanilla extract

A pinch of salt

¼ cup unsweetened coconut milk

1 ½ cups water

½ cup ice

Preparation:

1. Blend spinach and water first.

2. When smooth, add oats, vanilla extract, salt, coconut milk, and ice and blend until fully mixed.

3. Pour right into a tall glass and serve.

Variation:

If you're not drinking this smoothie immediately, you can take away the ice cubes in the ingredients and simply chill inside the refrigerator to cool off the drink before serving.

Smoothie fact:

Coconut milk is a superb weight loss option to other styles of milk as the medium-chain essential fatty acids it includes are absorbed rapidly by your body and burned as fuel rather than being stockpiled as fat.

Pineapple and Coconut Spinach Smoothie

Yield: 1 glass

Ingredients:

1 cup spinach

2 cups pineapple chunks

¼ cup of coconut milk

½ cup of water

½ cup ice

Preparation:

1. Place all ingredients inside a blender. Blend until mixed thoroughly.

2. Pour right into a glass and serve immediately.

Variation:

To get a chunkier smoothie, substitute coconut milk with ½ cup shredded coconut.

You can even use romaine lettuce or any other mild green vegetable rather than spinach

Smoothie fact:

That is a refreshing smoothie that packs in dietary fibers, antioxidants, and vitamins A and C. Each serving contains only 110 calories and 21 grams of carbohydrates.

Nice Lettuce Punch Smoothie

Yield: 1 glass

Ingredients:

1 cup romaine lettuce

½ cup fresh strawberries

½ mid-sized banana

½ apple (cored and chopped)

¼ cup dried apricots

1 tablespoon ground flaxseeds

½ cup nondairy milk

½ cup ice

Preparation:

1. Blend lettuce, strawberries, and milk until mixed thoroughly.

2. Add banana, apple, apricot, and flaxseed. Whiz on broadband until smooth.

3. Blend in ice last.

4. Pour right into a tall glass and drink while cold.

Variation:

Pre-soak apricots before blending for your smoother blend.

Supply ½ cup of oats for a far more filling alternative.

Smoothie fact:

Romaine lettuce is wonderful for your heart. It is abundant with beta-carotene and Vitamin C that it's good for avoiding the accumulation of cholesterol in your heart's arteries. The folic acid in lettuce helps repair weakened arteries, as the potassium it includes helps lower blood circulation pressure.

Because romaine lettuce includes a slightly bitter taste, it is advisable to blend it with sweet fruits when coming up with a smoothie.

Lovely and Sour Green Smoothie

Yield: 2 glasses

Ingredients:

¼ cup broccoli florets

¼ cup cauliflower florets

½ pink grapefruit

½ tablespoon linseeds

½ tablespoon almond nuts

2 tablespoons dried pitted dates (pre-soaked for any smoother blend)

½ cup dried apricots

½ cup nondairy milk

1 cup of water

Preparation:

1. Put water, milk, broccoli, cauliflower, and grapefruit within a blender.

Whiz until mixed thoroughly.

2. Put linseeds, almonds, dates, and apricots. Blend until smooth.

3. Pour right into a tall glass and revel in.

Variation:

If you discover the taste of grapefruit too sharp for the liking, you might substitute it with equal part orange to get a sweeter taste.

Add more normal water if you discover your smoothie quite thick.

Green Smoothie Bowl with Mango + Hemp Seeds

Author: Sherrie Castellano | With Food + Love

Prep period: 1 min

Cook time: 1 min

Total time: 2 mins

Serves: 1 bowl

If you don't have hemp seeds or cannot source them, flax seeds work also. The very best part about smoothie bowls will be the toppings. Discover notes below for more topping choices. This recipe makes 1 bowl, and it could easily exist double or tripled.

Ingredients

1 banana

1/2 cup mango, diced

3 handfuls baby kale or spinach

2 tablespoons

1/2 cup unsweetened almond milk or preferred milk

1/8 teaspoon

handful of ice

Instructions

Combine all the ingredients inside a blender and action until totally smooth.

Pour the smoothie right into a bowl and layer around the toppings. Here I used sliced mango, a drizzle of honey, hemp seeds, and red Russian kale sprouts.

Snickerdoodle Green Smoothie

Serves 1

1 handful spinach

1 frozen banana

1/2 small avocado

1/4 cup unsweetened almond milk

1/2 tsp vanilla

1/4 tsp cinnamon

Blend until creamy and smooth!

Note: If you don't possess a higher-powered blender, you should use 1/2 cup of almond milk!

Green Warrior Protein Smoothie

Not only is it an entire protein source, but hemp hearts also support the ideal balance of omega 3-6-9 essential fatty acids and are saturated in fiber. They work wonderfully to make this smoothie super creamy, all without needing any banana. If you need a sweeter smoothie, experience absolves to swap the grapefruit juice for coconut water or orange juice, or put in a touch of liquid sweetener.

Ingredients:

1/2 cup (125 mL) fresh red grapefruit juice*
1 cup (25 g) destemmed dinosaur/lacinato kale or baby spinach**
1 large nice apple (200 g), cored and roughly chopped
1 cup (130 g) sliced cucumber
1 medium/large celery stalk (85 g), chopped (about 3/4 cup)
3 tablespoons (30 g) hemp hearts, or even to taste

1/3 cup (55 g) frozen mango

2 tablespoons (4 g) packed fresh mint leaves

1/2 teaspoons (7.5 mL) virgin coconut oil (optional)

4 ice, or as needed

Directions:

Juice a red grapefruit and add 1/2 cup grapefruit juice towards the blender.

Now add the kale (or spinach), apple, cucumber, celery, hemp, mango, mint, coconut oil (if using), and ice. Blend on high until super smooth. (If utilizing a Vitamix, utilize the tamper adhere to push it down until it mixes). You can include a little bit of water if essential to obtain it blending. Pour right into a glass and revel in immediately! This makes enough for big glass with some leftover and that means you may also divide it into two portions and save one for later.

Nutrition Information

Tips:

* Feel absolve to sub the grapefruit juice with orange juice or coconut water in case a sweeter smoothie is desired.

VEGAN MANGO-COCONUT GREEN SMOOTHIE

PREP: five minutes TOTAL: 5 MINUTES

Using its light coconut milk base - no dairy here - this vegan green smoothie is completely creamy and coconutty. Mango gives it a tropical vibe that means it tastes just like a trip to the beach.

INGREDIENTS:

1 cup fresh washed spinach leaves, packed (I generally use packaged, pre-washed baby spinach)

1 cup fresh or frozen mango cubes

1/2 medium banana

3/4 cup light canned coconut milk (can substitute almond milk, however, the result is probably not as creamy and won't taste coconutty)

1/2 cup orange juice

1/2 cup ice

OPTIONAL ADDITIONS:

1 tablespoon coconut butter (this adds a little more coconut flavor plus fiber and just a little protein)

1 tablespoon ground flaxseeds (these then add more fiber plus omega-3 essential fatty acids and just a little protein)

Chopped mango or coconut for topping

DIRECTIONS:

Place all ingredients within a blender and puree until smooth. Pour into glasses, add toppings if desired, and serve to have a straw.

Low-Carb Shamrock Protein Smoothie

Ingredients (makes 1 serving)

1/2 average avocado (100 g/ 3.5 oz)

1/4 cup coconut milk or heavy whipping cream

1/4 cup fresh spinach

fresh mint or mint extract to taste

1/4 cup vanilla or simple whey protein or egg white protein powder (Jay Robb) or collagen powder or plant-based NuZest (25 g/ 0.9 oz)

2 tbsp pistachio nuts (unsalted) (20 g/ 0.7 oz)

seeds from 1/2 vanilla bean or 1 tsp sugar-free vanilla extract

3-6 drops liquid Stevia extract or another healthy low-carb sweetener out of this list

1/2 normal water and optionally ice

Instructions

Wash the mint and spinach, halve and peel the avocado and blend until smooth with all of those other ingredients. Serve immediately.

Tropical Green Smoothie

prep time: five minutes

total time: five minutes

We promise this healthy green smoothie doesn't taste healthy whatsoever! It tastes just like a virgin piña colada that simply is green and healthy.

INGREDIENTS

2 cups frozen spinach

1 cup frozen pineapple chunks

1 cup frozen mango chunks

1 medium ripe banana, peeled (previously frozen in chunks is ideal)

1 cup strawberries, blueberries, raspberries, or perhaps a favorite berry, optional

1 cup milk (cow's, almond, soy, coconut, kefir, horchata)

1 teaspoon vanilla extract

sweetener, to taste (sugar, agave, stevia, honey, maple syrup, Medjool dates)

INSTRUCTIONS

Place all ingredients inside the canister of the Vita-Mix or blender and blend until smooth and creamy. Serve immediately.

Pour extra portions into freezer-safe cups and freeze for one month, thawing before serving (or microwaving for approximately 30 seconds)

NOTES

All ingredients and quantities are to taste. Use seasonal fruits or vary the levels of fruits, to taste. I take advantage of frozen fruit and prefer it to fresh since it keeps the smoothie cold, without adding ice which waters it down. Frozen is cheaper and I could buy in bulk and retain in the freezer and use it when needed.

Optionally, consider adding a scoop of protein powder, a dollop of yogurt for extra protein; add fat for stamina such as coconut oil, coconut butter, peanut butter, almond/cashew/sunflower seed/Cookie Butter. Blend with juice to improve the quantity of Vitamin C.

Put coconut flakes, nuts, seeds, dried fruits, or your preferred smoothie add-ins to either the blender canister before blending or garnish smoothie with them after blending.

The recipe is vegan (use vegan milk, avoid honey), gluten-free, soy-free, and nut-free as written. Be mindful any ingredients used and added optionally are ideal for your dietary needs.

Blueberry & Peanut Butter Green Smoothie

1 ripe banana

1/2 cups fresh spinach

1 cup frozen blueberries

1/4 cup yogurt (I used vanilla, basic or blueberry works too) splash of milk

1/2 tablespoon creamy peanut butter

1 tablespoon chia seeds

1. Blend all ingredients in a blender until smooth. Add more blueberries if you'd like your smoothie just a little thicker. Once smooth, add chia seeds and pulse many times. Enjoy!

Metabolism Boosting Green Smoothie

That is a twist on the classic green smoothie recipe. It's a spinach smoothie recipe which blends perfectly using the delicious flavors of strawberry and oranges (always a yummy combination).

The metabolism-boosting secret may be the almond milk, which contains extra protein and creaminess. Studies show that protein escalates the thermic aftereffect of food (TEF) because of the spare calories necessary to digest it. This causes growth in your metabolic process.

INGREDIENTS

1 orange peeled

⅓ cup strawberries

1 cup raw spinach

1 cup almond milk

INSTRUCTIONS

Add all of the green smoothie recipes ingredients to a blender.

Blend green smoothie until smooth, adding more water as a need to reach the desired thickness.

Serve, and wash out your blender immediately to avoid sticking.

Scrub Yourself Clean Green Smoothie

This is among the best recipes for any detox smoothie flush. Not merely will it taste delicious, but it additionally helps increase your metabolism, too!

Broccoli can be an extremely healthy vegetable, also known as a "super veggie". It's saturated in many nutrients, including vitamin C, vitamin K, fiber, potassium, and iron. Broccoli also includes even more protein than almost every other vegetables, gives you a supplementary metabolic boost.

This green smoothie cleansing recipe is ideal for someone who's not used to smoothie recipes for weight loss. The flavors are mild, as well as the nourishment is high.

INGREDIENTS

½ cup strawberries

¼ cup pineapple

1 cup broccoli florets

1 teaspoon honey

1 cup almond milk

INSTRUCTIONS

Add all of the green smoothie recipes ingredients to a blender.

Blend green smoothie until smooth, adding more water as a need to reach the desired thickness.

Serve, and wash out your blender immediately to avoid sticking.

Purple Passion Green Smoothie

INGREDIENTS

½ cup strawberries

¼ cup blueberries

1 cup raw spinach

¼ cup Greek yogurt

1 cup of water

INSTRUCTIONS

Add all of the green smoothie recipes ingredients to a blender.

Blend green smoothie until smooth, adding more water as needed to reach the desired thickness.

Serve, and wash out your blender immediately to avoid sticking.

Strawberry Banana Green Smoothie

INGREDIENTS

½ cup strawberries

1 banana

1 cup raw spinach

½ cup almond milk

1 teaspoon vanilla extract

INSTRUCTIONS

Add all of the green smoothie recipes ingredients to a blender.

Blend green smoothie until smooth, adding more water as needed to reach the desired thickness.

Serve, and wash out your blender immediately to avoid sticking.

Apple Pie Green Smoothie

INGREDIENTS

1 apple peeled and cored

¼ cup blueberries

¼ teaspoon cinnamon

⅛ teaspoon nutmeg

1 cup spinach

1 tablespoon chia seeds

1 teaspoon vanilla extract

1 cup of water

INSTRUCTIONS

Add all of the green smoothie recipes ingredients to a blender.

Blend green smoothie until smooth, adding more water as a need to reach the desired thickness.

Serve, and wash out your blender immediately to avoid sticking.

Electric Green Boost

That is a delicious green smoothie recipe that has a bright green color. It's filled with vitamin C because of the double dose of pineapple and oranges.

Pineapples certainly are a great way to obtain many nutrients, such as vitamin C, manganese, copper, and folate. Pineapples also include a plant compound called bromelain, which is connected with many health advantages, such as improved immunity, fighting cancer, faster wound healing, and better gut health.

INGREDIENTS

¼ cup pineapple

1 orange peeled

1 cup raw spinach

1 cup almond milk

INSTRUCTIONS

Add all of the green smoothie recipes ingredients to a blender.

Blend green smoothie until smooth, adding more water as needed to reach the desired thickness.

Serve, and wash out your blender immediately to avoid sticking.

Sweetie Pie Green Smoothie

INGREDIENTS

1 cup lovely peas

1 banana

½ cup blueberries

1 cup almond milk

1 tablespoon chia seeds

½ teaspoon honey

INSTRUCTIONS

Add all of the green smoothie recipes ingredients to a blender.

Blend green smoothie until smooth, adding more water as a need to reach the desired thickness.

Serve, and wash out your blender immediately to avoid sticking.

Mango Cucumber Green Smoothie

INGREDIENTS

¼ cup mango

1 orange peeled

1 cup cut cucumber

1 tablespoon flax seeds

1 cup spinach

INSTRUCTIONS

Add all of the green smoothie recipes ingredients to a blender.

Blend green smoothie until smooth, adding more water as needed to reach the desired thickness.

Serve, and wash out your blender immediately to avoid sticking.

Green Tropical Sunrise

INGREDIENTS

¼ cup pineapple

1 orange peeled

1 carrot

1 cup spinach

1 tablespoon flax seeds

1 cup of water

INSTRUCTIONS

Add all of the green smoothie recipes ingredients to a blender.

Blend green smoothie until smooth, adding more water as a need to reach the desired thickness.

Serve, and wash out your blender immediately to avoid sticking.

Kale Almond Milk Smoothie

If you're seeking to put more kale to your daily diet, this smoothie diet drink can help you do so… and ease any pain by using nature's ibuprofen: cherries.

EQUIPMENT
Blender

INGREDIENTS
½ cup cherries
½ cup blueberries
1 cup fresh kale
2 teaspoons honey
1 cup almond milk

INSTRUCTIONS

Add all of the green smoothie recipes ingredients to a blender.
Blend green smoothie until smooth, adding more water as a need to reach the desired thickness.

Serve, and wash out your blender immediately to avoid sticking.